The Long Covid Handbook

GEZ MEDINGER &
PROFESSOR DANNY
ALTMANN

PENGUIN BOOKS

PENGUIN BOOKS

UK | USA | Canada | Ireland | Australia
India | New Zealand | South Africa

Penguin Books is part of the Penguin Random House group of companies
whose addresses can be found at global.penguinrandomhouse.com

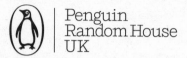

Penguin
Random House
UK

First published 2022
001

Typeset in 12/14.75 pt Dante MT Std by Integra Software Services Pvt. Ltd, Pondicherry
Printed and bound in Great Britain by Clays Ltd, Elcograf S.p.A.

The authorised representative in the EEA is Penguin Random House Ireland,
Morrison Chambers, 32 Nassau Street, Dublin D02 YH68

A CIP catalogue record for this book is available from the British Library

ISBN: 978–1–529–90012–5

www.greenpenguin.co.uk

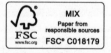

Contents

Introduction

In early March 2020, I was in the hills above Los Angeles – getting a suntan, trying to get my second feature film off the ground and training for my fourth marathon. The weather was delightful, my legs were strong, and I was confident of hitting my two hours fifty minutes target in the London Marathon the following month. The only problem was that somewhere in central China a pangolin had partied too hard with a bat, and now a pandemic was brewing.* The world – and my life – was about to change immeasurably.

I flew back to London on 6 March, and less than a week later had my first symptom – a peculiar nausea. The following day, chills and stomach upset. All the colleagues I'd shared a meeting room with a few days prior were ill too. There were no tests, so no one could be *sure*, but Covid was exploding across London.

My initial illness wasn't too severe. I was able to work a few hours a day and felt foolishly and quietly smug that my immune system was obviously better than my colleagues', who were feverish, coughing and having a general shocker. The London Marathon now looked like it was going to be cancelled, but I was so keen not to lose my hard-won fitness that in the second week of the illness I tried going for short jogs.

By this point my colleagues were recovering. I was confident that in a few days I'd be right as rain too. After all, the government was saying that if you didn't end up in hospital, then your isolation could end after a week, by which point you'd be fit to go back to work.

---

* The pangolin's role as the intermediate host that enabled the transmission of Covid from bats to humans remains conjecture. There is yet to be agreement among the scientific community on the origin of the virus.

Only I didn't get better. I kept running – going slowly, telling myself that it was only a matter of time – but the weeks went past and still I felt awful. And then, five weeks in, I felt it: a very specific 'grizzly' feeling in my throat and chest that I'd not experienced for twenty-two years. That feeling was the signature symptom of post-viral fatigue syndrome (PVFS), which I experienced for a year after being ill with glandular fever. *Oh God no*, I thought, *I can't be doing that for* another *whole year. Not now.*

So, I decided to make a film for my nascent YouTube channel to examine the potential links between the novel coronavirus and PVFS. Could it be possible that swathes of people would be struck down with a complex, poorly understood and often completely debilitating condition, even after a mild initial Covid infection? I wasn't sure if anyone would find their way to the film (especially given my paltry subscriber base at the time), but it gained an audience in the tens of thousands immediately – people all around the world, who were crying out for someone to recognise what was happening to them.

I thought I'd make only one film on the subject. But then I made another. And why not one more? *It'll be a trilogy*, I thought. And now here I am, more than two years and eighty films later. Still not back to where I was at in Los Angeles, running 20km at race pace every day, but able to live a busy life without relapsing every week as I did in the beginning.

The vast improvement in my quality of life has been due in large part to making myself Guinea Pig No. 1, incorporating every piece of expert advice and research accumulated on my journey into my own life to aid my recovery. Having made a lot of progress, my goal now is to share the lessons that I, and other recovered long haulers, have learnt – often the hard way.

I couldn't be more pleased to be collaborating on this project with Professor Danny Altmann, one of the UK's most respected immunologists and an expert on post-viral conditions to boot. Since early in the pandemic, he has been prepared to put his head above the parapet and speak on behalf of patients struggling to get recognition from the medical establishment. Danny is also running a large research project at Imperial College London that is investigating the role of immune system abnormalities and auto-immunity (which describes when our immune system attacks our own cells) in Long Covid, and so is at the very forefront of bio-medical understanding of the illness.

Between us, we hope to present a spectrum of the knowledge that exists at the time of writing – from the anecdotal experiences that I have observed in the Long Covid community through to my own patient-led studies and the hard science that's accumulating as more research, trials and publications reach the light of day.

Perhaps you're a Long Covid sufferer yourself, or a family member or partner of someone who is. Or perhaps you're a clinician seeing patients and looking for a resource that brings everything we know about Long Covid together. This is that resource. Danny and I have tried to make the knowledge, lessons and science herein as accessible as possible, because if anyone knows how difficult it is to absorb information with brain fog, it's someone with Long Covid.

We will break down the key topics into short chapters. Rather than present you with a solid wall of text, I will be your narrator, while Danny will break down the knotty and established science relevant to each topic in separate 'boxout' sections, like that below. At the end of most chapters, there is a quick Q&A with Danny and other key contributors, picking up some of the outstanding questions.

Like Gez, my introduction to the world of Covid also came in March 2020, when my research team opted to pivot from our 'day jobs' investigating infection and immunity to efforts at decoding immunity to severe acute respiratory syndrome coronavirus 2 (SARS-CoV-2), the virus that causes Covid. More than two years in, we have all become so expert in the topic that it's hard to think back to that time of a virtually blank canvas. Although I've spent my life researching the molecular immunology of pathways (i.e. how the body's immune system responds to infection) in a wide variety of bacterial, viral, fungal and autoimmune diseases, here was a new disease about which we knew nothing. Since that period, we've worked on Covid immunity pretty much seven days a week, publishing our findings in journals such as *The Lancet*, *Science* and *Nature*. Within a few months, one of my oldest friends who'd been infected early in that first wave gave me a detailed and accurate description of what was to become known as Long Covid. Previously an extremely busy, active person, she felt she'd had the wind knocked out of her, could barely walk around the block and felt constantly fatigued. This was vaguely familiar and alarming.

One of the flagship 'day-job' projects we'd had to suspend was a collaboration across clinical sites in Brazil, which aimed to establish why so many patients infected with the mosquito-borne chikungunya virus go on to develop a chronic, disabling illness that can drag on for years. One of our next papers, published in the *British Medical Journal*, was a kind of manifesto for the route forward to understand Long Covid. I'd always been quite motivated about the need to communicate about research with the public, press and policymakers. This communication began to seem really critical in a time of uncertainty and panic. No one wants to come across as a smart alec or mansplainer, but here was a situation in which you couldn't turn on the TV or radio without a politician expounding on 'antibodies' or 'herd immunity', topics that I'd lived and breathed from the first day of my PhD studies at the age of twenty-one. My diary began to fill up with daily sessions with journalists, TV crews, politicians and patient groups. During one of these sessions, I met Gez making one of his films. We've kept in close touch ever since, often exchanging news of the latest research findings. The Long Covid story is remarkable in the sense that the medical agenda has been driven entirely by patients themselves and their communication across social media platforms. I've met terrific, medically articulate people through those groups and acquired from them a crash course in living with this disease that now informs all our research. With that in mind, my aspiration here is to do right by people with Long Covid in trying to offer an honest and accessible distillate of all I've learnt and anything that could be helpful. The price I pay for this is that, while Gez's narrative will often come across as dramatic and exciting, I'm cast in the role of 'Professor Boring', as the voice of the medical establishment. It's a role I'm content to take if it offers useful illumination.

It will be self-evident from this book that Long Covid research is in its embryonic stage, sitting at an interface between the patient advocates and the medical research professionals. In that context it's hopefully useful that this book has two distinct voices from those different perspectives. The two views can inevitably become polarised at times. Gez has his role in drawing together the lived experience of the sufferers including their search for therapeutic answers. It is this clamour for answers that will in time wend its way into formal research studies. My career has drummed into me the paramount need to ignore anecdotes in favour of a laser-focus on the statistically-powered, controlled trial. That is, when hearing about 'evidence' in Long Covid, I set the bar in exactly the same place as if I were asked to peer review it for *Nature* or *The Lancet*. This means that sometimes Gez and I will not agree. I don't endorse every statement he makes, and vice versa. Long Covid has yet to achieve consensus so we see this breadth as a plus. It also means that my formality may sometimes annoy you – you may find that the hypothesis or treatment that seems most central to your view has received short shrift from me because it hasn't yet crossed that bar. Who knows, with time (and data) you may have the last laugh.

So, without further ado, let's begin.

CHAPTER 1: *What Is Long Covid?*

One of the hardest parts of trying to describe Long Covid is that it may be very different for you from how it is for me. But for almost all of us who experience it – long haulers, as we are sometimes known – the illness impairs almost every aspect of day-to-day life. Most long haulers are unable to socialise or work as they could before, they are most certainly unable to exercise as they could before and often they are even unable to eat and drink as they could before.

Other than some bags under the eyes, you might look pretty normal. Those around you – unless they've experienced chronic illness themselves – may struggle to understand what you're going through. Although perhaps that's not surprising: Long Covid comes with a bewildering array of symptoms – 203 of them, according to a patient-led study published by The Lancet Group.[1] Of course, no one experiences all 203 of these symptoms. The Covid lottery is something of an (un) lucky dip. Long Covid can encompass a single symptom such as anosmia, through to the more common cluster of multiple (usually around 5–20) symptoms. The term is also applicable to someone with a known complication after Covid-19, such as a stroke or severe lung damage. This book won't take a dogmatic stance on the duration of persistent symptoms that count as a Long Covid case – both 4 weeks or 12 weeks from start of infection have been applied. Since many do improve significantly from 4–12 weeks, the latter cut-off is useful for demarcating those set on more of a 'long-hauler' trajectory.

> **What is Long Covid in a single sentence?**
> Long Covid is a long-term consequence of SARS-CoV-2 infection, lasting beyond the initial 'acute' phase of infection, affecting multiple bodily organs and systems, causing a huge variety of symptoms and of varying severity and duration, potentially relapsing and remitting over time.

Crucially, long haulers' symptoms are not likely to be consistent. They vary from week to week, day to day, even minute to minute. Day-to-day tasks and planning even as far ahead as tomorrow are difficult when you have no idea how you'll be feeling at any point in the future.

Long Covid is debilitating by nature. People who haven't experienced fatigue, the most common symptom of Long Covid, often imagine it to be close to the feeling of tiredness after heavy exercise or an extremely long day. Before the pandemic hit, if you'd asked me, I would have said I knew what spending every last drop of energy felt like too, as someone who'd run several marathons and ran my own business, frequently putting in consecutive all-nighters.

But the systemic exhaustion that Long Covid deals up is on an entirely different level – perhaps only familiar to those with severe chronic illnesses, such as myalgic encephalomyelitis, also known as chronic fatigue syndrome (ME/CFS). This exhaustion really needs a new word to describe it, because 'fatigue' doesn't do it justice. In my patient-led research, this 'fatigue' is repeatedly cited as the most crippling symptom for long haulers across the board. Fatigue is exhaustion down to your very bones. Even simple activities like reading or watching TV are too much, let alone the absurd idea of being able to hold a conversation.

One American study compared 1,295 Covid long haulers with 2,395 patients with cancer, and in the process found that the long haulers were roughly *twice* as likely to self-report poor physical health or pain as those with cancer.[2] Of course, while fatigue might be the most frequently reported, there's over 200 other symptoms which, on any given day, might knock you for six.

The symptoms

Without making an exhaustive list of all 203 symptoms, here are some of the most common:

- fatigue
- brain fog (aka cognitive dysfunction)
- chest pain or tightness
- insomnia

- heart palpitations
- dizziness
- joint pain
- depression and anxiety
- tinnitus and earaches
- nausea, diarrhoea and stomach aches
- headaches
- skin problems (peeling, rashes, itching)
- continued loss of taste and smell.

But there's no end of unusual stuff being reported by long haulers, from the profoundly disabling to the merely 'upsetting', such as:

- hair loss
- tingling and numbness
- nerve pain
- menstrual changes
- erectile dysfunction
- urinary incontinence
- blurred vision
- hallucinations.

If you've got more than one of these symptoms (for the first time) and have recently had Covid, then it's possible you're suffering from Long Covid. As you may have gathered, there's very little correlation between the symptoms you might have experienced in your acute infection and those you could experience in Long Covid, which can present in almost any system of the body.

And, in the UK at least, where so many people did not have access to Covid tests early in the pandemic, clinicians can now diagnose the condition without needing evidence of infection – or, for that matter, a diagnostic test. Because, at the time of writing, a reliable, easily accessible test that proves you have Long Covid does not exist.

Historically this absence of 'testability' has contributed to poor understanding of post-viral conditions. It's simply too easy to write off the symptoms as stress, anxiety or burnout, which has happened to innumerable people with ME/CFS and Lyme disease for decades.

Long-term effects of Covid-19[3]

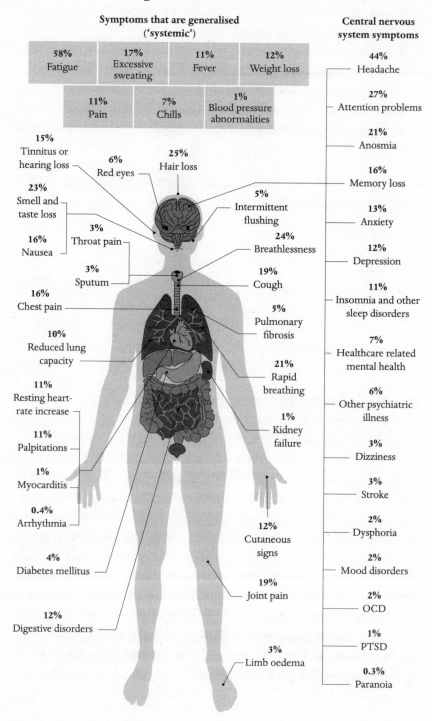

Symptoms that are generalised ('systemic')

58% Fatigue	17% Excessive sweating	11% Fever	12% Weight loss
	11% Pain	7% Chills	1% Blood pressure abnormalities

Central nervous system symptoms

44% Headache

27% Attention problems

21% Anosmia

16% Memory loss

13% Anxiety

12% Depression

11% Insomnia and other sleep disorders

7% Healthcare related mental health

6% Other psychiatric illness

3% Dizziness

3% Stroke

2% Dysphoria

2% Mood disorders

2% OCD

1% PTSD

0.3% Paranoia

15% Tinnitus or hearing loss

6% Red eyes

25% Hair loss

5% Intermittent flushing

23% Smell and taste loss

3% Throat pain

16% Nausea

24% Breathlessness

3% Sputum

19% Cough

16% Chest pain

5% Pulmonary fibrosis

10% Reduced lung capacity

11% Resting heart-rate increase

21% Rapid breathing

11% Palpitations

1% Kidney failure

1% Myocarditis

0.4% Arrhythmia

12% Cutaneous signs

4% Diabetes mellitus

19% Joint pain

12% Digestive disorders

3% Limb oedema

From a clinical and academic perspective, what's different or interesting about Long Covid?

Modern medicine is meant to be about preventing painful and debilitating disease. We're grappling with a new virus which, depending on which estimates you use, has caused at least 5 million deaths so far. The World Health Organization recently upped the estimated global death toll to 15 million in May 2022.

Yet in medicine, we don't just count deaths, we count symptoms and quality of life. So, there's actually a much larger number of people who are affected in the long term by a chronic disease that impairs their life on a day-to-day basis – whether it's their ability to function normally, work normally or even get out of bed in the morning.

You can't easily quantify it, and it is often assigned less importance than death, but the point I've often made is: let's just suppose that in an ideal world our vaccines work so well that we cease to worry about intensive care units (ICUs) being overrun and a daily death toll. We might still be talking about this pandemic in terms of the Long Covid impact for years to come, long after we're worrying about trying to deal with the acute disease.

What's particularly challenging is that, as we learn more and more, it's impossible for any one doctor or clinician to understand absolutely everything about modern medicine. It takes a lifetime just to get your head round everything we know about the immune system, for example.

So, we get increasing degrees of specialisation, and knowledge gets siloed. You have specialists for each organ system or different parts of physiology. But the problem with Long Covid is that it doesn't, in most cases, neatly fall into one or two of those silos. It seems to involve all of them, and thus is outside the remit of any one conventional specialist.

More to the point, Long Covid defies easy testing. Recent research has suggested that low cortisol levels (a hormone responsible for regulating stress response and suppressing inflammation) may be implicated in Long Covid and could at some stage form part of a diagnostic test, but there is yet to be widespread agreement on markers that indicate severity or what might be going on. It's even possible that a single diagnostic test might not ever be developed for such a heterogeneous disorder.[4] Solving the question of what Long Covid actually *is* seems to me to need a helicopter view at the same time as a deep dive. How in the current system do you do both simultaneously?

What's the solution to this need for both a deep and broad understanding of Long Covid, given the constraints of the current medical system?

It's unbelievably challenging. One of the things that happens is that, in any professional specialty, we always think that we're better, more knowledgeable and better trained than the previous generation, and also that 'the youngsters don't know what they're talking about'.

The perennial whinge of the older generation is that the young doctors of today have been so shoddily trained that they barely understand their own specialty and are terrified of seeing anybody outside it. But, to understand complex diseases, you do need to understand the whole person and you need an excellent command of general internal medicine.

I often compare Long Covid to lupus. Let's say you're a doctor sitting in your clinic and the medical textbook chapter on lupus had never been written. A patient walks in – let's say it's a young woman who doesn't know what to do because she's got a skin rash. Maybe if you were clever or empathetic you'd refer her to a dermatologist and you'd think, *Wow, that was a bit tedious.*

Then she comes back three months later for a repeat appointment. Her rash has cleared up, but she has incredible respiratory problems and tells you that she can't walk up hills any more. You think, *Last time she said it was her skin, this time she says it's her lungs. Is she attention-seeking? What's going on with her?* So perhaps you refer her to a respiratory team. Three months later she turns up again and says she's having trouble walking because her joints are really playing up. Now you're perhaps wondering if this could be psychosomatic, but you refer her to a rheumatologist.

Perhaps you can see where I'm heading with this. You might assume that the woman was an attention-seeker unless you understood lupus and the fact that there's a common mechanism underlying all the symptoms she had. And, of course, this person wasn't making it up. She had a bona-fide autoimmune disease called systemic lupus erythematosus, which merits a multi-system, multi-organ, multi-specialty treatment approach.

So, at the end of my laboured metaphor, I think that's where we are with Long Covid. People have diverse symptoms that are remitting and relapsing, coming and going. Some people are being empathetic, whereas others are thinking, *Are they making it up?* because we haven't yet written the textbook chapter on Long Covid. While there's still a long way to go, I'd like to think we're making progress and that perhaps this book can help fill some of the knowledge gaps.

Scientists and clinicians are using fancy, high-tech tool kits to figure out how Long Covid works at a functional, cellular level. In the end, the devil is in the detail, and we're quite good at measuring detail. I'm optimistic that it won't take too long until we understand Long Covid as well as – or maybe even better than – we understand lupus.

No matter how tired, exhausted and sick you may feel right now, or how hard it is to get through paragraph after paragraph, Danny's optimism is merited, despite what people with other post-viral conditions have experienced for the past twenty or thirty years. More on the reasons for that optimism a little later. But right now, let's stay on topic. That was symptoms. Now let's address *phenotypes*.

The phenotypes

Some questions to get us going. If you look at everyone with Long Covid, is there a pattern around the grouping of symptoms? For example, why might you have joint pain and shortness of breath, while I have headaches and palpitations?

Are there lots of people who have these same combinations of symptoms, and if so, what could that tell us about how the disease works? Is it possible that understanding these groupings and what causes them could help people avoid Long Covid altogether? It is these groupings of symptoms that we call *phenotypes* – literally, how the disease process looks.

These are huge, important questions that medicine hasn't quite answered yet. But research is ongoing that might shine some light on the answers.

> **How easily can we demonstrate phenotypes of symptoms for Long Covid?**
> I think the jury is still out, simply because you can look at it in so many different ways.
>
> In medicine we tend break it down into the 'lumpers', who are attempting to understand the whole of this disease, and the 'splitters', who slice the disease into an infinite number of thin little slices.
>
> Until you've got a clear picture of the disease mechanism (i.e. how exactly the disease produces symptoms on a physiological level), trying to delineate phenotypes is always a bit like putting the cart before the horse. You say to yourself, 'I've got to simplify my question, so I'm going to look only at patients who report mainly respiratory symptoms – the people who can't have any kind of exertion and permanently feel breathless.'

And it then might be useful to say, 'Let's look at the respiratory folk who are predominantly experiencing breathlessness compared to the neuro folk who are predominantly troubled by brain fog and word-finding problems.' I have a feeling that if I tried to do that, I might be bombed out of the water by people saying, 'Well, I'm both' or 'I'm respiratory but the respiratory symptoms only came after my joint and skin problems.'

It might turn out that my categories are a load of nonsense, because you can't get the answer until you've got the answer.

Some of the large research projects to date[5, 6] have clustered Covid long haulers into the following groups based on the severity of the initial infection:

- mild disease, not hospitalised
- hospitalised
- admitted to ICU.

But when it comes to understanding the disease, these groupings can only take us so far. For one, the vast majority of long haulers out there fall into the first category. Furthermore, those in the third category – people who were admitted to the ICU – are more likely to be experiencing the effects of organ damage than the potentially more diverse drivers of Long Covid in others. So ultimately we will need a finer level of categorisation by symptom clusters to determine mechanism and then develop effective, ideally individualised treatments.

This finer categorisation is coming, with recent research (using huge volumes of data from the ZOE app) suggesting certain symptom clusters.[7] However, based on what I've observed in more than two years embedded in the community and from surveying thousands of long haulers in my own patient-led research, I would like to propose some phenotypes which might help us when it comes to treating and managing symptoms. If we break down the first category of 'mild disease, not hospitalised' in terms of symptoms, I would argue three main groupings have emerged:

- increased intolerance to foods, allergies, headaches, skin issues, breathing problems and gut issues
- brain fog, fatigue, post-exertional malaise (i.e. a worsening of symptoms after physical, mental or emotional activity, commonly known as PEM) and cognitive exhaustion
- increased heart rate (palpitations), nausea, dizziness (especially on standing), insomnia, anxiety, chest pain, vision problems and irregular temperature regulation.

Now, you might have symptoms from all three groups! That isn't uncommon *at all*. But what seems to be the case is that long haulers' conditions are predominantly led by one group of symptoms, which respond particularly to one set of triggers – or indeed treatment. The symptoms in the first grouping, for example, might be related to mast cell activation.

What is mast cell activation syndrome?

Mast cells are a type of immune cell found all over the body. Some investigators suggest that some Long Covid symptoms might be related to what is known as mast cell activation syndrome (MCAS). The limits of symptoms that could have an MCAS-like origin is a source of controversy among allergy/immunology/dermatology experts. For example, many lung problems following Covid-19 have other known or likely mechanisms other than MCAS. In MCAS, mast cells are hyperactivated, which leads to excessive release of histamine. In Long Covid, this histamine potentially operates via the same immune pathways that are up-regulated in people with conditions such as asthma, eczema and food and dust allergies to cause some of the symptoms discussed above.

If you've ever experienced allergies (such as hay fever) before, or have had eczema or asthma, then the chances of your Long Covid experience being influenced by something related to MCAS may be high.[8] The symptoms mentioned are by no means exclusive – MCAS can present in many different ways, from disrupted gut function to aching joints, skin problems and shortness of breath.

The second group of symptoms might be related to metabolic dysfunction. In simple terms this means that the chemistry that produces energy in your body's cells has been affected. One of the most interesting theories proposed so far suggests that this metabolic dysfunction might be due to a deficiency of nicotinamide adenine dinucleotide (NAD+).[9, 10] NAD+ is a co-enzyme that's critical in the creation of adenosine triphosphate (ATP), which powers just about all our cellular function, and neural, muscle or other tissue.

A deficiency of NAD+ leads our body to use alternative metabolic pathways that are less efficient, leading to the symptoms mentioned in the second grouping (again, this list is most definitely not exclusive!).

The third group is perhaps the most common symptom cluster in Long Covid: symptoms potentially related to dysautonomia and postural orthostatic tachycardia syndrome (PoTS). Dysautonomia can be thought of as malfunctioning of the autonomic nervous system, which is normally responsible for the regulation of bodily functions such as heart rate, digestion, breathing, balance, temperature, blood pressure and more.

PoTS is defined as an increase in your heart rate by thirty beats per minute or more when you sit or stand up. It is related to dysautonomia and very common in long haulers.[11] It might not sound like much on paper, but it can be incredibly disabling, leaving people bedbound and able to move only short distances. Climbing a flight of stairs can feel like attempting to summit Everest for some people with PoTS.

Many long haulers report a combination that resembles mast cell activation, metabolic dysfunction and autonomic dysfunction in greater or lesser proportions. Each of the conditions has different treatment and management strategies, and how well you respond to those treatments could suggest what your personal balance of them might be.

We will discuss why you might have your particular blend of symptoms in the next chapter. If you're desperate to jump ahead to those treatment or management strategies, then you'll be wanting chapters 9 and 10. I wouldn't blame you!

How can people 'prove' that they have Long Covid?
Sadly, we're now in a phase when improved clarity on the definition of Long Covid is becoming ever more critical. The premise throughout much of this book has been that no un-equivocal diagnostic criteria exist, and that in many regards they are superfluous, as long haulers are in little doubt about their changed health status following SARS-CoV-2 infection. Medical professionals with an interest in Long Covid are well aware of the urgency and continue to work hard to define and refine a consensus working definition.[12]

However, we are hurtling into a brave new world in which interpretation of Long Covid diagnostic criteria will become the stuff of daily disputes at employment tribunals and dis-ability benefit assessments, as well as being questioned by pension providers and health insurers. This is in addition to the more basic requirement to clearly define cases for health-care referrals into treatment pathways and for healthcare budgeting purposes. Clear diagnostic definitions will also be crucial for defining entry and stratification in clinical trials.

For my taste, notwithstanding many plausible academic articles and their press releases that have passed across my lap-top claiming to fill this need for a diagnostic test, we are simply not there yet. It is possible to have full-blown, bona-fide Long Covid either with or without PCR proof of infection, or evi-dence of detectable antiviral antibodies. According to WHO criteria, the requirement is a clinical picture compatible with having had Covid-19. Only a small minority of people infected with SARS-CoV-2 have undergone any type of imaging or scans. However, enough data has already been gathered to be sure that it is possible to have persistent Long Covid symptoms without having any visible end-organ damage seen on routine imaging. Conversely, it's possible to have organ changes visible in scans but to have no persistent symptoms.[13, 14]

As researchers race to identify reliable biomarkers to be the basis for a consensus laboratory test for Long Covid, we need an interim, internationally agreed working definition. Until we can do better, a working definition can be accrued from comparison with health status before infection, evidence in support of having had Covid, and then evidence of newly persistent symptoms from the Long Covid list. At the other end of the process, we also need much more clarity on reporting of symptom changes to facilitate analysis of clinical trial outcomes.

GEZ: How similar is Long Covid to other long viral conditions, such as long chikungunya or PVFS (post-viral fatigue syndrome) after glandular fever or other viruses?

DANNY: It's another unwritten medical textbook chapter. I can't think of any book I've ever seen written on post-viral syndromes, or any medical school lectures that have ever been given on the topic because it hasn't been a thing.

I might try to pull it all together and write something about it soon, because I'm someone who really likes infectious disease and also really likes autoimmunity. I've previously looked at chikungunya virus and autoimmunity, Ebola virus and autoimmunity, herpesviruses and autoimmunity – and now at Covid and autoimmunity.

It's really hard to pull together any common denominators, but the simplest place to start is to ask: 'What is autoimmunity?' Auto-immunity is the breakdown of immunological tolerance so that the immune system does something that it's not meant to do, which is to start recognising and responding to your own tissues, your own proteins.

There is a whole branch of medicine dedicated to post-infectious autoimmunity, so most doctors would recognise the existence of reactive arthritis, for example: this is the idea that you could have salmonella food poisoning and then come down with joint disease.

So, at least we've got a starting point of being able to link an infection to an autoimmune consequence. But when it comes to commonalities between long viral conditions after Ebola, chikun-gunya, glandular fever and Covid, we just don't know enough yet.

GEZ: The closest other viral infection we've got to compare Covid with is severe acute respiratory syndrome (SARS), which was caused by a similar coronavirus. Are there any academic papers out there on the long-term consequences of that?

DANNY: Yes, a few, and we need to dig them up. But unfortunately, with the benefit of hindsight, it's clear that for both SARS and Middle East respiratory syndrome (MERS) we should have done the homework and the follow-up so much better.

With SARS and MERS, the acute emergency came and went and was dealt with. So many of the questions that should have been addressed afterwards haven't been. But there's a small number of quite decent papers on the long-term consequences of SARS that look very much like what we're talking about here.[15] So, that's a big deal: an almost identical virus and almost identical consequences.

GEZ: How easy is it to track down the patients who were reviewed in those initial follow-up studies one to three years after having SARS?[16] Seeing how they did subsequently would almost be like seeing into the future for those with Long Covid now.

DANNY: There absolutely was a persistent, long-Covid-like syndrome after SARS and MERS. There was no funding and no pressure to look at it. It's only with hindsight that people are looking at it now. The best hope is probably the cohort in Singapore, who have undergone quite a lot of immunological testing, as well as the healthcare workers who were infected in Toronto. To some extent, those people are indeed our crystal ball into the future for Long Covid. I recently managed to make contact with one of the consultants who treated the Toronto patients during the 2002–04 outbreak there and followed them up for many years. The outlook he described was rather discouraging. There's quite a large caveat, which is that this isn't really a like-for-like comparison with the global Long Covid caseload. All the consultant's patients were hospitalised with their initial infections and so their chronic symptoms developed from a baseline with an element of post-traumatic stress disorder.

Summary

Long Covid is a very long way from some people's perception of it as 'being a bit out of sorts'. The condition can't be easily categorised and can be extremely severe, impacting on people's quality of life in multiple, highly debilitating ways. Long Covid can vary from hour to hour, day to day and week to week, and new symptoms can appear months into the experience. For most people, it will be an illness unlike any other they've ever had, which raises the question you've been thinking about for months: *why me?*

CHAPTER 2: *Who Gets Long Covid and Why?*

If you've been dealing with Long Covid, whether for months or years, at some point you've probably thought, *why me?* We've all looked at the people who got Covid at the same time and wondered why they bounced back to full health in a week or two, when we didn't. What's different about us?

This is actually a very profound question, and a comprehensive answer would likely reveal the full pathology underpinning the condition. Unfortunately, we're not quite able to fully answer it yet, but we're starting to see studies published in high-profile journals like *Nature Communications* and *Cell* that identify certain risk factors for developing Long Covid.[1,2]

Who is more likely to get Long Covid?

Several studies have looked at large cohorts of thousands or hundreds of thousands of acute cases of Covid (the initial week or two of infection, from which most people recover) to see which individuals went on to develop Long Covid.[3-5] The following characteristics emerged as being statistically associated with an increased risk of Long Covid:

- hospitalisation during acute infection (and particularly admission to the ICU)
- high number of symptoms during acute infection
- female sex
- higher-than-average body-mass index (BMI)
- asthma
- poorer baseline health (indicated by a high number of other pre-existing conditions).

These associations were based on statistical analysis of a large number of cases. Thus, there are clearly many people with Long Covid who do not have any of these risk factors, and may indeed have excellent baseline health.

One of the challenges with large data samples like these is that there are frequently distortions due to the nature of data collection in the early days of the pandemic, when for the most part only people who were hospitalised got a PCR test (and thus were included in these samples). Many of the 'mild' cases in the community in early 2020 (including me) went on to develop Long Covid without ever having had a positive test. (The quotation marks around 'mild' are necessary – for many of us the experience didn't feel mild at all!) Thus, there is a huge community subset (who arguably account for the majority of people with Long Covid) who do not appear in these statistics.

What we're looking at then in these figures is perhaps an indication of the *damage* done by the virus, as opposed to the *disease engine* (my term for describing the 'things going wrong in the body' that cause symptoms) of Long Covid. It seems like these might be two different things. Those who were hospitalised have organ damage commensurate with the severity of their acute infection, whereas 'mild' acute cases may go on to develop severe Long Covid without necessarily having any visible organ damage under magnetic resonance imaging (MRI) investigation. So, the cause of symptoms in these two groups (i.e. the 'disease engine') might be different, yet both groups might currently might be considered to have Long Covid. This is a necessary distinction that is rarely made in the scientific literature or by the media. Early published papers on Long Covid tend to focus on the first group (those who were hospitalised during the initial infection), whereas my patient-led research tends to reflect the second ('mild' acute cases that did not require hospitalisation).

Why are these risk factors associated with Long Covid?
Looking at the words most frequently mentioned in the abstracts (summaries) of the research papers published to date,[6-10] the most common is probably 'female'. Then you'll see terms like 'middle-aged', 'asthma', 'post-menopause', 'EBV reactivation' and 'high BMI'. Age and high BMI are associated with an increased probability of being hospitalised in the acute phase of Covid infection.

I think we have to be careful about how we group these risk factors, lest we create more rather than less confusion. High BMI being a risk factor likely relates to the fact that people with high BMI are more likely to have been hospitalised with severe Covid. In terms of Long Covid history and symptoms, we may come to think of the group hospitalised with severe Covid as quite distinct from the person with Long Covid who is more likely to be younger, female and to not necessarily have a raised BMI, or to have been hospitalised. The object of this distinction is not to infer any judgement about the different groups, but rather to acknowledge that we may have a way to go in sorting out stratification of Long Covid 'phenotypes' (clinical causality and appearance) in a way that will really be useful for treatment pathways and clinical trials.

However, some elements of these findings make sense in terms of what we know about the condition at the moment. Long Covid certainly looks like other conditions characterised by autoimmunity and immunopathogenesis (diseases that result from some part of an immune response). Women have a much higher propensity for developing autoimmune disease – this is true of relatively common autoimmune diseases like rheumatoid arthritis or lupus, for example. One of the reasons for this is that the immune system interacts strongly with the endocrine system (which governs your hormones). The key difference between sexes are the endocrine cascades. All those hormonal differences you learn about in biology class don't just affect secondary sexual characteristics (armpit hair and breasts in women, beards and deep voices in men, for example), they also feed into many of the nuances of immune programming. It is fair to say that this seems to lead to differences in immune regulation between sexes, and women tend to have more 'activatable' immune systems.

Asthma seems to be a genuine risk factor for Long Covid. Let's go back a step to explain why. Much work over recent years has been devoted to defining the genetics and immune programming that predisposes someone to asthma. People who have asthma walk around for their whole lives with what could be called skewed immune programming at one end of the allergic (sometimes called 'atopic') spectrum – such that their immune system overreacts to certain triggers. By describing people at one end of this 'allergic spectrum', we simply mean the ones who may be generally more prone to the type of immunity that can underpin anything from pollen or animal-fur allergies, to food allergies and eczema. One theory to explain why people have such immune programming is the so-called hygiene hypothesis, which argues that our immune systems evolved over the millennia to deal with a particular kind of pathogen and parasite load – particularly in the gut. This type of immunity is generically called 'Th2 immunity'. It's a rather aggressive form of immunity, useful if you need to be able to expel a tapeworm from your gut.

Nowadays, though, most people in high-income countries don't have any parasite load at all. So, we're walking around with a completely inappropriate immune program that's ready to be pushed over into inappropriate Th2 responses. This is what causes what are known as 'atopic' diseases like asthma, eczema and hay fever, which affect around 20% of the population in Western countries. Several studies now suggest that people with atopic conditions are more likely to get Long Covid.[11-13]

Finally let's talk about Epstein-Barr virus (EBV), which, during acute infection, is also known as infectious mononucleosis or glandular fever. EBV is a herpesvirus that normally sits latent in the blood cells of people who have been infected with it – think of it as hibernation. One of the key findings in the *Cell* paper was that the presence of *reactivated* EBV in the bloodstream during the acute Covid episode predicted an increased likelihood of developing Long Covid. The finding that EBV reactivation could play a role in Long Covid is exciting to me because scientists have spent decades talking about latent EBV reactivation and what it means. It has been hypothesised to be implicated in various autoimmune diseases, and the publication of this paper in *Cell* coincided almost to the week with the most impressive paper that's ever been published on the subject (in *Science*, another high-profile journal). The *Science* paper reported the results of a huge study of EBV, which suggested that the virus plays a role in causing multiple sclerosis (MS).[14] This link has been debated for several decades.

EBV is a very different kind of virus from SARS-CoV-2. Most of us get it at an early age. As mentioned above, in most people it then sits dormant inside a particular type of white blood cells called B lymphocytes (the cells that make antibodies). Most people will be positive for EBV and not know it, but you'll also have heard the stereotypical story of the teenager who goes off to university, discovers snogging for the first time and then comes down with debilitating glandular fever. In those cases, the patients' immune systems are disrupted, and they can't function normally for up to a year or more – finding it hard to study, let alone party, and becoming prone to every passing bug and sniffle.

There are some real similarities with Long Covid. You can have a very mild acute phase or a highly symptomatic one, but either way it can have real long-term consequences. Trying to figure out why and when EBV causes symptoms can feel a bit like watching arthouse cinema: you spend a lot of time asking, 'Why did that happen then!?' It comes and goes variably in different people with very different amounts of virus in their system.

The discovery of the links between EBV and both MS (with an extremely high probability) and Long Covid gives us a great starting point to dive in deeper with future research.

One of the other findings of the *Cell* paper was that patients who had a high viral load in the acute phase of their Covid infection were more likely to develop Long Covid. While perhaps this isn't surprising – it might even seem logical – it could also explain the huge number of long haulers who were 'created' in the first wave in February–March 2020. In Western countries, there were no mitigation measures for controlling the spread of disease at the time – no social distancing, no face masks, no indoor ventilation and no vaccines. Thus, the initial viral dose causing infection in many cases might have been huge.

Further exploration of viral loads could perhaps offer some clues about the various disease mechanisms implicated in Long Covid. Since SARS-CoV-2 is a virus that damages and kills infected cells in target organs such as the lungs, heart and brain, leaving a trail of scarred tissue and inflammation in its wake, a simple explanation would be that people with more virus in their system for longer might be more likely to develop Long Covid. But in fact this explanation points more towards the organ damage 'disease engine' that we see in hospitalised cohorts, who often have a different presentation of symptoms from those 'mild' cases in the community I mentioned earlier. Long Covid clearly cannot be simply correlated just with how much virus was around, as some of the most severe cases of Long Covid occur in people who had mild or even asymptomatic acute episodes.

The *Cell* paper also suggested that the presence of certain auto-antibodies (antibodies that mistakenly attack the body's own cells) was correlated with the likelihood of developing Long Covid. But before we discuss this, it would be helpful to take a closer look at what autoimmunity actually is.

What is autoimmunity?

What gets immunologists out of bed in the morning is the grand question: 'What's the immune system all about?'

The immune system recognises things that shouldn't be inside your body or that suggest that something dangerous is going on in your body. When this happens, the immune system activates enormous – and potentially damaging – inflammatory pathways via T cells and B cells (types of white blood cell that fight pathogens), so that you can get rid of the stuff that shouldn't be there. These pathogens might be worms, viruses, fungi, tumours or bacteria. As humanity evolved, our bodies didn't necessarily pre-emptively produce receptors that could specifically recognise Ebola virus, for example. Rather, they produced millions of receptors, with the hope that at least one of them would recognise the virus. That's how the immune system has always worked, in every organism on the planet.

The catch is that the immune system identifies potential threats by their shape, which can be quite similar to the shapes of proteins and chemicals that our own bodies produce. As a result, sometimes our bodies confuse these naturally occurring chemicals with threats, which produces an immune response against ourselves. Immunologists refer to our immune system's ability to recognise our own bodies and not attack them as self-tolerance. When the immune system does get confused, there are lots of fail-safe mechanisms in place to delete autoimmune repertoires, whether B cells or T cells,

---

so that most of the time, most of us don't develop auto-immune diseases.

But sometimes errors of self-tolerance can occur, and your immune system recognises bits of your own body as if they were something dangerous and produces an inflammatory-damaging response to them. In many diseases, the result is that autoimmune antibodies attack parts of your own body, such as in lupus, thyroiditis, rheumatoid arthritis (to some extent), myasthenia gravis and various forms of nephritis and kidney disease. In extreme instances such autoimmune diseases can result in organ damage and death.

Patient-led research

The papers published to date provide clues about what might be going on physiologically in Long Covid and open up avenues for future research, but in my experience they don't necessarily reflect what the community sees around them in terms of who is unlucky enough to suffer.

SEX DISTRIBUTION

Published studies with huge datasets have shown women are more frequently affected by Long Covid than men.[15, 16] And indeed, one of the most obvious correlations between the data from my patient-led studies and the published data is this finding. In my various studies, women have accounted for anywhere between 70 and 86% of the patient group.

As with any data sample, there are some caveats to bear in mind in terms of how selection bias can affect the data collected. The recruitment for my studies happened largely on social media platforms, including Facebook, Twitter and Slack. Most respondents came from a selection of international Long Covid support groups on Facebook. There is likely to be a bias in terms of the sociocultural demographic that uses these groups and these platforms, and this bias will have an effect on the reliability of the data. For some of the data collected, this bias is likely to be relevant; for other data it might be much less important. With regards to the finding that more women than men are affected by Long Covid, it is possible that women are more likely to use the online support groups and to take part in research like mine. Therefore, the actual proportion of women affected (relative to men) could be lower than my data suggests. However, pretty much all the data that has been published suggests a similar sex breakdown in the patient population, so I don't think the bias is too great. The lower bound of my data (i.e. 70% women, 30% men) seems to reflect the patient group as a whole, no matter the setting.

ACTIVITY LEVEL

Unlike some of the clinical studies, which at the larger end of the spectrum have included only a few hundred patients (the study of the data provided by the ZOE app is a notable exception[17]), the sample size of my groups was also larger – often between 1,500 and 2,000 respondents. My feeling is that this data is a better representation of Long Covid in the community than was often seen in the early clinical studies, when often only patients who had been hospitalised during their initial Covid infection were recruited to participate. In chapter 5 we'll address why these mechanisms of Long Covid might be different.

But back to the activity level. In the first of my large studies, which had 1,859 participants, I found that two-thirds of people with Long Covid were previously highly active (exercising vigorously at least three times a week).[18] This is a slightly higher proportion than found in the general population. Only 3.8% of participants were not physically active. So, we were looking at a fit slice of the population who were being affected by Long Covid – not necessarily the same demographic who were at risk of severe illness in the acute phase (commonly understood to be people who were of advanced age, had severe underlying conditions or were immunocompromised).

What's the link between fatness, fitness and immune function?

You could write a whole book on this topic. There's an enormous amount of research on the interface between immunology and metabolic disease. In people who have large deposits of adipose tissue (fat), this tissue can become a depot for poorly programmed immune cells, which can be pro-inflammatory and can predispose people to several metabolic diseases, notably type 2 diabetes.[19]

However, being fit is not necessarily good for your immune system either. People who do a lot of physical training produce corticosteroids, which can suppress immunity. This is one of the reasons why runners often get ill the week after a marathon. The relationship between arduous exercise and susceptibility to infection has been long debated, particularly in the field of sports medicine. Among elite athletes, infections are a close second to sports injuries as a contributor to days lost from sport.[20]

AGE PROFILE

The next most striking finding in my data was the age profile of the long haulers surveyed. Although almost all age groups were represented, the thirty-five to forty-four and forty-five to fifty-four categories were three times more likely to appear among respondents than other 'ten-year' age brackets. This 'bulge in the middle' has been replicated in every single one of my studies to date, no matter which aspect of Long Covid I was researching. Again, it is possible that selection bias may be playing a role (children, gen Z and people over seventy use the platforms where I recruited my participants less frequently) but these findings do seem to reflect cases in the community. Anecdotally, while older members of society may have managed their risk of exposure and caught Covid in lower numbers than those in middle age, the same cannot be said of millennials, university students and children. So, what's going on?

How does our immune system change as we age?
Our immune systems change throughout life. Children have large, active thymuses, the organ that acts as mission control for educating and directing T cells, one of the key agents of the immune system. As you grow into adulthood, the thymus shrivels up to almost nothing and puts out far fewer T cells. Thus, as you get older, you have fewer new T cells and more 'exhausted' T cells, which have gone through lots of cell divisions and are less functional and more damaged as a result.

Another autoimmune condition that displays the 'bulge in the middle' age profile noted in Gez's Long Covid dataset is new-onset rheumatoid arthritis. This similarity between the two conditions is extremely interesting and important.

IMMUNE CONDITIONS

The potential association between autoimmunity, other immune conditions and Long Covid was suggested relatively early in the pandemic, so I included a line of relevant questioning in one of my studies in November 2020, to investigate which conditions – if any – might be risk factors.[21]

My approach was simple: I measured how many people in my sample were affected by each autoimmune condition before their Covid infection, and then compared the prevalence in my sample to that in the general population. If a higher proportion of people were affected by a disease in my sample, then that could suggest that the condition was a risk factor for developing Long Covid and could give us some clues about the disease mechanism underpinning Long Covid.

The first condition that I looked at was type 1 diabetes, in which the body's immune system attacks and destroys the cells in the pancreas that produce insulin. In the UK, 2.6 million people have diabetes, and about one in ten of these people have type 1 diabetes. This gives us a prevalence of 0.6% in the population. (For reference, 62% of the participants in my study were from the UK, so using UK data for comparisons seemed the most sensible, and anyway the prevalence of the conditions I was exploring is broadly similar across Western nations generally.) Of my sample of 824 long haulers, only three had type 1 diabetes. To save you getting your calculator out, that equates to 0.4% of the study sample – a similar prevalence as in the general population. For those of you who are curious types, there were seventeen people with type 2 diabetes in the sample (in the general population there are around nine people with type 2 diabetes for every person with type 1). So, whichever way you spin it, diabetes didn't seem to be a risk factor for Long Covid in this study's population.

The next condition that made sense to investigate was rheumatoid arthritis. Not to be confused with the more common osteoarthritis, which is caused by wear and tear of joints, rheumatoid arthritis is an autoimmune condition and can affect adults at a range of ages. Figures for the frequency of the disease in the general population are easy to find – the prevalence is 0.44% in men and 1.16% in women.[22] It's interesting to note a similar sex distribution to what we see in Long Covid. Balanced to the sex distribution of my sample, I would have expected to see a prevalence of rheumatoid arthritis of around 0.9% if the disease was *not* associated with the probability of developing Long Covid. However, 115 people among my sample of 824 had rheumatoid arthritis – equating to 14%, fifteen times higher than we'd expect if the disease was not a risk factor for developing Long Covid. Considering Danny's comments about the age profile similarity between Long Covid and rheumatoid arthritis in the last boxout, this link would be one of my top picks for future research. Are some of the same autoantibodies involved in both Long Covid and rheumatoid arthritis? If I were a betting man, I'd definitely have a little flutter on that one.

How about that nefarious triangle of asthma, hay fever and eczema – known collectively as atopic conditions? As Danny described, these conditions are largely associated with inappropriate Th2 immune responses (which are often triggered by various allergens). Data for the proportion of the UK population that has an atopic condition is hard to come by, but if we add together figures for the prevalence of the individual diseases, we can estimate that roughly 30.5% of people have at least one of asthma, hay fever or eczema. Of course, some people might have two or all three of these diseases and so will be counted in the data multiple times. Fortunately, I can use my own data as a model to establish how many people have more than one of the triumvirate and apply that to the nationwide figure. Looking at how many people in my cohort have more than one atopic condition (and assuming this is similar in the general population) would suggest that our expected atopic percentage of the population is 22.2%.

So, against this expected figure of 22.2%, how many of our 824 long haulers experienced at least one of asthma, hay fever or eczema prior to their Covid infection? The answer is 473, or 57.4%. This is a highly striking difference by any measure. However, we do need to compensate for the fact that only about 38% of cases of asthma are associated with atopy (i.e. the remainder of cases are caused by something other than Th2 immunity).[23] When we remove people with non-atopic asthma from the sample, the prevalence of at least one atopic condition falls to 52.8% – still more than twice the proportion in the general population. This finding tallies with the previously discussed association between Long Covid and asthma reported in other studies and gives us plenty to go on, in terms of understanding both the possible mechanisms of disease and which treatments might be effective. We'll address the related topic of MCAS in chapter 5.

POST-VIRAL FATIGUE SYNDROME (PVFS)

The final risk factor I wanted to investigate was previous post-viral fatigue syndrome (PVFS). If people have already had their socks knocked off for months or years after other viral infections, might that increase their risk of developing Long Covid? First let's consider the levels of PVFS we might expect to see in the population at large. Between 2001 and 2013, the annual incidence of PVFS was 12.2 cases per 100,000 people in the UK.[24] We've got some maths to do though to turn that into an expected proportion that we can compare against our sample. The average age of people in our sample was forty-five. PVFS is only really diagnosed in adulthood. Let's be generous and say that the average person in our group had thirty-five years (since they were ten) to appear in this kind of statistic. That gives us an expected prevalence of people who previously had PVFS of 0.4%. By contrast, a whopping 23% of our sample reported previous PVFS. It's worth acknowledging that the quoted statistics that give us our general population figure of 0.4% are probably on the low side, as it represents only formally *diagnosed* cases, and the condition frequently goes undiagnosed. However, with my data suggesting that the prevalence of previous PVFS was sixty-two times higher in people with Long Covid than in the general population, it would take a vast underestimate in the general population figure for this result not to be extremely interesting.

There are a couple of other associations that could be important among the Long Covid community, but they are difficult to quantify and evaluate. So, at this stage, we move into the next level down of our evidence base, where the connections are more speculative.

Anecdotal risk factors

In the two and a half years that I've been in the Long Covid community I have spoken to hundreds – possibly thousands – of other long haulers. Each of them has in turn spoken to many more. One of the other traits that seems to be disproportionately common among the patient population is some kind of connective tissue disorder. Rheumatoid arthritis fits into this category, as do Ehlers-Danlos Syndrome, hypermobility spectrum disorders and fibromyalgia. Previous research has noted a connection between some of these disorders and ME/CFS,[25] and so far anecdotal evidence suggests a similar link with Long Covid.

Moving on to some more controversial territory, previous trauma of some type and what might be unscientifically termed type A personalities (i.e. people who could be described as work-aholics, outgoing, ambitious, organised and impatient) also seem to be common in the Long Covid population. Now if you've been around the ME/CFS community for some time, bear with me before immediately reaching for the red buzzer. Both of these two traits have previously been cited by the biopsychosocial lobby to support their argument that the origin of ME/CFS is *psychological*. For a complete takedown of this point of view, turn to chapter 5 to read about the biological pathways implicated in Long Covid (and ME/CFS) or chapter 7 to learn more about the PACE trial, considered by many to have been discredited and debunked.

So, where am I going with this? We know that people with post-traumatic stress disorder may be more likely to develop autoimmune disease, which suggests that trauma can have a physiological impact on the body (for more on this see chapter 9).[26] To understand how this in turn can affect behaviour, we need to turn to the autonomic nervous system.

What is the autonomic nervous system?
At the simplest level, the autonomic nervous system is the part of the nervous system that operates automatic bodily functions – things like heart rate, breathing, digestion and temperature control. It is divided into two parts: the sympathetic (which is involved in the 'fight-or-flight' response) and the parasympathetic nervous system (whose functions are sometimes summarised as 'rest and digest' or 'feed and breed').

The American neuroscientist Stephen Porges elaborates further on the autonomic system in what he terms the 'polyvagal theory'.[27] It has to be pointed out that this hypothesis still remains firmly in the scientific realms of theory rather than accepted medical phenomenon, but to those of us with Long Covid the polyvagal theory makes a lot of empirical sense. In addition to the polyvagal theory being just that – a theory – we also don't yet have *evidence* published in academic journals to link it to Long Covid. We are simply too early in this journey for that, but I believe it is worth including because of the remarkable way it lines up with long haulers' experiences, and the implications it raises for managing symptoms (see chapter 9).

Porges adds a further state, 'immobilisation', to the traditionally understood parasympathetic response (i.e rest and digest). He then creates a hierarchy between immobilisation, the traditional parasympathetic response and the sympathetic response (i.e. fight or flight). Imagine a set of traffic lights, where in this hierarchy the 'safe' state (parasympathetic response) resides at the bottom in the place of the green light. The next state up is termed 'mobilisation' (sympathetic response) and can be imagined as the amber light, representing the cues of threat or danger, or chronic stress. The final stage is called 'immobilisation', which corresponds to the red light and represents the shutdown of the body, a 'freeze' state in which the focus is purely on survival and very little active function is possible.

This state of immobilisation is probably one that sounds familiar to everyone who's had Long Covid. It is where we inevitably end up after spending too long in a state of sympathetic nervous system response. In fact, many of the symptoms of Long Covid can be attributed to autonomic dysfunction, leading us to spend an inappropriate amount of time in 'fight or flight' and not enough in 'rest, digest and heal'.[28, 29]

But what is happening physically when this is going on? During the state of immobilisation, Porges argues that the dorsal branch

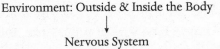

Porges's View of the ANS

Environment: Outside & Inside the Body

↓

Nervous System

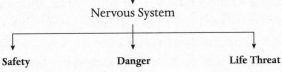

Safety	Danger	Life Threat
• Regulated and relaxed	• Fight or Flight	• Immobilisation
• Parasympathetic System	• Sympathetic Nervous System	• Parasympathetic System
• Ventral Vagal Pathway	• Hyperarousal	• Dorsal Vagal Pathway
• 'Social Engagement System'	• Ready to move away from what we	• Survival State
• We connect and engage	perceive as dangerous	• Shame, hopelessness, overwhelm
• We're ready to learn, attend and problem-solve	• Faster breathing, blood pressure increases	• Hypoarousal
• Deep breathing, slow heart rate	• Dissociative rage, panic, quick to blame, attack, judge	• Dissociated collapse
• We communicate well		• Shutdown
		• 'Freeze'

of the vagus nerve (which is the main component of the parasympathetic nervous system) enacts the shutdown. In addition to affecting the function of the heart and lungs, the dorsal branch affects how our body functions below the diaphragm, with knock-on effects on the gut. So, when you're in immobilisation expect physiological changes too, with less frequent trips to the bathroom as your gut function slows down.

So, how are previous experiences of trauma connected to this polyvagal theory? I spoke to clinical psychologist (and fellow long hauler) Dr Sally Riggs about it. She suggested that if you have a history of trauma, then it is quite possible that you've spent most of your life between the states of flight or fight and immobilisation. One of the consequences of this is that feeling 'safe' can actually feel 'scary', because it's unfamiliar, uncomfortable and not 'natural'. If you consider the polyvagal hierarchy, then the route back down to safety from immobilisation at the top has to take you through the 'danger' stage. For example, Dr Riggs describes how she's observed long haulers undertake activities like deep breathing or yoga, which are often considered to be soothing. However, in some cases they can seem to prompt sympathetic nervous system symptoms which are uncomfortable and overwhelming for the body. What happens then is an immediate shutdown that sends you straight back to immobilisation.

As far as established science is concerned, the polyvagal theory remains just a hypothesis. It does, however, make a lot of sense to me, especially in terms of understanding why some of us might develop Long Covid. My argument would be that people who spent disproportionate amounts of time with their autonomic systems *under stress* – however we want to define that – are more likely to then find that a Covid infection tips this autonomic system over into full-blown dysautonomia.[30]

What is dysautonomia?

Dysautonomia has been much cited in studies of people with Long Covid. It describes the dysregulation of autonomic nervous system function and can present as a fast or slow heart rate, postural problems on standing, breathlessness, fatigue, headaches, anxiety, gastric issues or sleep disruption. A specific diagnosis that's often mentioned is PoTS (as discussed in chapter 1), which is caused by an abnormal autonomic response to the need to redistribute blood around the body. This state of 'orthostatic intolerance' (intolerance of standing upright) involves activation of the vagus nerve in response to standing, which can lead to tachycardia (high heart rate), low blood pressure, dizziness and fainting.

As with other aspects of Long Covid, people have described at least two mechanistic pathways that could link the condition

---

to this PoTS disease profile: viral infection could cause direct cellular damage to the autonomic nervous system, or auto-antibodies targeting the receptors that are involved in many aspects of normal parasympathetic function could be produced in response to the infection.

We are now, fortunately, at the stage when it is becoming widely accepted by the medical community that dysautonomia is one of the key symptom drivers in Long Covid, with the classic symptoms of dizziness, racing heart rate and headache also accompanied by sympathetic nervous system overdrive. Unfortunately, however, curative treatments for dysautonomia are limited, and most of the steps you can take revolve around management of the condition.

GEZ: Does vaccination reduce your chances of developing Long Covid?

DANNY: It seems to reduce it – some studies say by about half[31] – but the risk remains very real. Overall, I'd say I've been terribly saddened by the devastating new Long Covid cases that have continued to pile up, even in the post-vaccination period. If you'd asked me to predict, I'd have guessed that Long Covid would have been largely a legacy of the severe, pre-vaccination waves through 2020. The fact that cases have continued to accrue since then in a largely vaccinated population shows just how little we really understand about the causes and immune regulation of Long Covid. The UK has acquired well over a million additional Long Covid cases in the post-vaccination Delta to Omicron period. Surely, that's perplexing.

GEZ: Does having Long Covid affect immunity against reinfection?

DANNY: Some long haulers have reported multiple infections. This has become one of those questions that has become difficult to answer in the era of Omicron: reinfection is terribly prevalent. In theory, it would be possible to collect the data allowing one to ask whether long haulers are more or less likely than others to be reinfected. It would be important to control for all the many variables: different initial infecting variants, different doses and types of vaccines. My suspicion is that the long haulers may show similar reinfection rates to others.

GEZ: Can you develop Long Covid after a reinfection, when you recovered fine after the first infection?

DANNY: Yes, anecdotally. Not developing Long Covid the first time is no guarantee you won't next time. There aren't studies on this yet, though. One of the obvious problems of living through this pandemic is that it throws new research questions at us in real-time, so much faster than we can set up research to find answers. You might perhaps imagine that mechanisms and phenotypes of Long Covid might look a little different in the distinct immune setting of reinfection. Also, Delta and Omicron, being such distinctive viruses when compared to the ancestral strain, might cause somewhat differing Long Covid. It's still too early to know.

GEZ: The paper in *Cell* found that the presence of certain autoantibodies was associated with the probability of developing Long Covid.[32] Am I right in thinking that these autoantibodies are not present in healthy people?

DANNY: You'd think that that would be a really straightforward question, but unfortunately it's not quite so simple to answer. Covid has provided the biggest human immunology dataset that anybody has ever studied, but there are enormous biases in the data, due to so many people having had an infection. We're finding all these exotic things but we don't really have a pre-Covid dataset to compare these observations against. Some French researchers published convincing data that some people with Covid make very damaging anti-interferon autoantibodies (which interferes with how cells protect themselves from invaders), but we don't know how many people might produce these autoantibodies in the absence of Covid.[33] Nevertheless these autoantibodies are a bona-fide marker of Covid severity. The other point raised by screening for autoantibodies (that my lab has mirrored in our research) is the discovery of lupus autoantibodies in people with Covid.

GEZ: Does that mean that lupus shares some pathophysiology (disease process or cause) with Long Covid?

DANNY: To answer this, it might help to explain what lupus is. Lupus is a moderately common autoimmune disease in which the body starts to make autoantibodies to both DNA and DNA–protein complexes. Of all things, DNA is the one that you really don't want to have an autoimmune response to because it's in every cell in your body. As a result, the autoantibodies come in many different flavours and specificities and have incredibly diverse impacts – that's why lupus affects the central nervous system, kidneys, lungs, joints and blood vessels. When you think of Long Covid, this sounds rather familiar, doesn't it?

GEZ: What's different about what we know about Long Covid at the moment and what we know about lupus?

DANNY: For lupus, we've never made enormous headway in identifying any infectious agents – unlike Covid, obviously. Lupus is also very ethnically skewed: in clinics in the UK and the USA, lupus is more commonly seen in young, Black women. And it's a sledgehammer, it's very severe. If lupus is not managed effectively, it can seriously damage your organs. We're not really seeing that level of severity in Long Covid, even without treatment.

GEZ: Is there anything we can see right now that differentiates Long Covid from lupus in terms of an autoimmune signature?

DANNY: Professor Alex Richter's team in Birmingham have been working on autoantibody tests, and the range of autoantibodies seems much broader and more diverse in Long Covid than in lupus.[34]

GEZ: So, still many more questions remaining on this front! In summary, though, is it fair to say that we're seeing a significant degree of autoimmunity in Long Covid?

DANNY: I think that's a fair statement, yes. It's certainly part of the story.

GEZ: You earlier spoke about how extremely fit people can suppress their immunity through steroid production, but it seems like what's happening in Long Covid is the opposite. When I take corticosteroids, my symptoms subside.

DANNY: Well, it could be to do with the way your body handled the virus – how receptive you were to it when it came in, or what kind of immune response you had when first infected. This response would have been affected by where you sit on the physical fitness spectrum, because people at the opposite ends of that spectrum definitely have different immune systems. Who's to say what the perfect immune system is to grapple with a new virus that we haven't seen before?

Summary

As with just about all factors surrounding Long Covid, the science is still developing when it comes to understanding who is at risk of the condition. But we are starting to see some trends validated with data. If you were to distil *all* the evidence (and anecdotal observations) for predisposing factors into one fictional character, they would look a little like this: Elsie is female, aged between thirty and fifty, and previously lived an extremely active, full-on life. She's not very good at taking breaks or slowing down. She has a history of mild asthma and had glandular fever when at university. Now, of course, not everyone will look like Elsie, but if she were a friend of mine I'd be advising her to take it *very* easy in the weeks after a Covid infection. This brings our discussion of who gets Long Covid and why to a close. But one huge and important subpopulation deserves its own chapter, and that comes next.

CHAPTER 3: Can Children Get Long Covid?

Early in the pandemic it was widely believed that children weren't affected by the novel coronavirus. This was because relatively few children needed to be hospitalised during the acute phase of illness. Then the identification of a small number of children with Covid who developed symptoms similar to those of Kawasaki syndrome (a rare disease in which blood vessels are inflamed by immune activation) suddenly made the international press. As time has gone on, the symptoms that these children experienced become known as paediatric multisystem inflammatory syndrome (PIMS), or multisystem inflammatory syndrome in children (MIS-C) in the USA. PIMS is quite rare, occurring in less than 0.5% of paediatric Covid cases.[1]

What has received rather less coverage in the media, and very little research funding, is the presentation of Long Covid in children. Just how many children are affected by Long Covid remains unclear. A wide range of estimates have been published in the scientific literature, from 1% of those who had an acute Covid infection at the lower bound, up to 25% in a recent meta-analysis of 80,071 children and adolescents.[2,3] The disparity in these estimates is probably due to differing methodology and selection criteria for which symptoms are considered by the researchers to constitute Long Covid, and whether a positive PCR test is required to qualify patients for inclusion. Whichever way you spin it, even if Long Covid only occurs in 1%, that's still a huge number of children, given that UK data suggests that most children have had Covid.[4]

One of the reasons that people may have been slow to recognise Long Covid in children is the continuing misapprehension, dating from the first wave of the pandemic in early 2020, that Covid is primarily a problem for the elderly. Each variant has affected different parts of the population and resulted in different symptom profiles. So, while the initial wave was dominated by discussion of care-home outbreaks, by the time we shifted from Alpha to Delta and then to Omicron and beyond, the pandemic had become one driven via spread in schools.

Official statistics in the UK suggest that 119,000 children and adolescents currently have Long Covid, 21,000 of whom have had it for at least a year. The Omicron wave was so pervasive in schools that recent Office for National Statistics (ONS) data estimated that over 1.5% of all children in the country have Long Covid.

And what about children who develop PIMS during the acute phase of infection? I talked with Sammie Mcfarland, founder and CEO of the charity Long Covid Kids. Sammie is a long hauler herself, and her daughter has had Long Covid symptoms for more than a year. In Sammie's experience, children with PIMS are often discharged from hospital and classified as having recovered, but in reality they often still have severe symptoms and soon find their way to Long Covid Kids for help. So, essentially, children who continue to have symptoms post-PIMS have Long Covid.

What does Long Covid typically look like in children?

Although Long Covid can manifest in as many perplexing different ways in children as in adults, there are a few symptoms that could be grouped into a typical paediatric presentation.[5] Unsurprisingly, the most common symptom is fatigue – just as it is in adults. Then there's insomnia, cognitive dysfunction, dysautonomia, anxiety and gastrointestinal disturbance, also not unfamiliar among the adult population. Then we start to branch off with symptoms that are more specific to young people: joint, nerve and abdominal pain, migraines, swelling, skin rashes, temperature dysregulation and sensory overload. Many children find overstimulation, whether auditory or visual, difficult to tolerate. Loud or intense sounds can be very difficult for children with Long Covid. Another frequent occurrence noted by Sammie is that children with Long Covid demonstrate large degrees of regression. One reported instance is that of a seventeen-year-old who had scholarships for further study, who, after getting Covid, spent all their time in their room playing with their Sylvanian Families toys from when they were six years old. This kind of story seems hard to believe, but the severity of Long Covid can lead to emotional coping mechanisms of this scale. The regression can also present in a number of different ways, including regressive behaviour around the rest of the family and relationships.

In extreme cases, children can have such difficulty swallowing and tolerating food that they end up being tube-fed.[6-8] In Sammie's experience, once children begin to be tube-fed, they are (so far) unlikely to go back to eating normal food. She also reports that some children with Long Covid experience extreme muscle weakness and struggle to stand unaided. Even after intensive physiotherapy, the improvements in some of these children are only minor. Sammie also raises reports of children who've become mute since getting Covid. This is a harder symptom to verify as it could be a result of the psychological pressure of the illness rather than a physiological problem. Either way, the impact is just as severe.

What do we know about long-tail viral conditions in children and adolescents?

While post-viral conditions have been identified in children before, Long Covid is quantitatively and qualitatively in a whole different ballpark. That's our starting point: no matter the age group, Long Covid is different. There's only really one virus relevant to children or adolescents that's comparable in terms of impact and that's EBV.

EBV plays an important part of the story of human evolution – you might say it's our oldest foe.

Coronaviruses, like those that cause the common cold, are generally thought of as fairly temporary infections – quick in, quick out. Herpesviruses, such as EBV, couldn't be more different. They tend to persist latent in the body, often for a lifetime. Herpesviruses were the first viruses associated with human cancers and are an incredibly successful, almost ubiquitous pathogen.

Before the advent of modern medicine, most of the planet was walking around with EBV in their throat, with parents passing that exposure on to their children. Nearly all of those infections were asymptomatic. Children grew up and went through their lives latently and persistently infected, and most of the time nobody cared. There are rare examples in which EBV is hugely important – it has been associated with some cancers, including lymphomas and nasopharyngeal carcinoma – but it's only in recent years that we've been able to make that connection.

Nowadays, there are whole cohorts of adolescents who reach adulthood and still test negative for EBV (potentially due to the increase in protective parenting behaviours). Then, as a result of lifestyle or environmental changes – such as moving away to university – they get exposed to the virus. The resulting illness is what we call glandular fever or infectious mononucleosis.

Glandular fever is one of the very few conditions in this age group that presents similarly to Long Covid. People with glandular fever experience fever, malaise and swollen lymph nodes, and are fatigued for a protracted period. So, even though EBV is different from SARS-CoV-2 in many ways, there are some very interesting commonalities. People have been researching the impact of glandular fever on the immune system in quite granular detail for decades. Some of the findings from that research could help to shed light on potential pathological mechanisms in Long Covid.

In one of my favourite studies of EBV, which was done by Professor Kristin Hogquist's research group at the University of Minnesota, new students at the university were tested for the virus.[9] Of these students, 37% had never had EBV. During their studies, nearly half of this group of students subsequently tested positive for EBV. The researchers were able to assess in real time how many students developed symptoms, how many remained asymptomatic and how many developed full-blown, persistent glandular fever, and drilled down into the differing immunological profiles of those groups.

To cut a long story short, when you do all the fancy immunological investigation in those groups, you build up a picture that seems rather like our direction of travel for Long Covid. For example, if you were to ask, 'Was the severity of EBV infection correlated with how much virus students had on board or the extent of their immune response?' (pertinent and familiar questions in the context of Long Covid), the answer would be a bit of both. Severely affected patients often started off with a high viral load and initially produced slightly poor antibodies against the virus, but then ended up with massively expanded populations of persistent T cells – sometimes even years later. These T cells were dominating their entire immune systems, almost to the exclusion of everything else, sometimes forming significant majorities of all lymphocytes in the blood, which to an immunologist is just extraordinary. If you've been following the science on Long Covid, this might sound familiar.

Long Covid in children and adolescents[10]

Cardiorespiratory
- Respiratory symptoms
- Sputum/nasal congestion
- Orthostatic intolerance
- Exercise intolerance
- Chest pain
- Rhinorrhea
- Cough
- Chest tightness
- Variations in heart rate
- Palpitations

Gastrointestinal
- Abdominal pain
- Constipation
- Diarrhoea
- Vomiting/nausea

Dermatologic/ Teguments
- Excessive sweating
- Dermatologic (dry skin, itchy skin, rashes, hives)
- Hair loss

Neuropsychiatric
- Mood (sad, tense, angry, anxiety, depression)
- Fatigue
- Sleep disorder (insomnia, hypersomnia, poor sleep quality)
- Headache
- Cognition (confusion, impaired concentration, learning difficulties, memory loss)
- Dizziness
- Neurological abnormalities (pins and needles, tremor, numbness)
- Balance problems

Others
- Loss of appetite
- Altered smell
- Body weight changes
- Muscle aches
- Altered taste
- Tinnitus, earache or vertigo
- Eye problems (conjuntivitis, dry eyes, problems seeing/blurred vision, photophobia, pain)
- Swollen lymph nodes
- Fever
- Changes in menstruation
- Urinary symptoms
- Speech disturbances

What are the challenges for children with Long Covid?

The fact that Long Covid is mostly an invisible illness only adds to the complex manifestations and its impacts on one's life. Now imagine that you're a child, who has yet to have the chance to develop the life skills or coping mechanisms of adulthood. Children or teenagers are still learning who they are. They haven't had a career and don't have any savings or insurance policies to claim against. They rely for support entirely on their parents, who may not understand the many complex manifestations of their illness or how difficult it can be psychologically. Across almost every support group on social media, adult long haulers have reported challenges in their relationships with their spouses or partners, but at least adults are more likely to be able to self-support to a greater extent. This is just the beginning of how hard it is for children and teenagers with Long Covid.

GOING TO SCHOOL

The charity Long Covid Kids estimates that 85 to 90% of children and adolescents with Long Covid routinely have to miss school. In the UK, there are very few provisions for those unable to attend school.* In many cases, unless you can manage classes designed for healthy students, you simply don't get educated. There are several reasons why kids with Long Covid might not be able to go to school: their fatigue could be too severe (even the travel there may be too exhausting, let alone the school day), their mobility too impaired or their concentration span too limited – and that's before we even get to the potential social stigma.

Some children with Long Covid might have parents who can afford to be off work and at home to help with their education, which could enable them to convalesce effectively. But many

---

* There is nominally a home tutor option available, but the process is incredibly difficult to navigate.

parents do not have that luxury. Furthermore, some parents might not believe in Long Covid, or the children's schools may even hound the parents and threaten prosecution unless their kids attend (which is happening in the UK, according to Long Covid Kids). Often, Sammie reports, children will try to go to school and push through, but subsequently relapse – it's the classic 'boom and bust' that adult long haulers will identify with. The consequential negative effects on the children's recovery is very real, as is the impact on their education.

SOCIALISATION

Children's social groups are complex at the best of times. When chronic invisible illness is added to the mix, they become even more so. Often, the affected child's friends will ask 'When are you coming back?' for perhaps two or three months. Then the question becomes 'Well, you don't look that ill, why aren't you coming back?' Following that, there's a degree of anger, then bullying, then stigma – when the child simply becomes ignored.

One of the biggest challenges for kids with Long Covid is that they struggle to stay awake in the evening when their friends are on social media. They might have no one to interact with during the day when their friends are at school and their parents are at work. It might be important to factor in the level of embarrassment, depending on the age group involved. Embarrassment is probably less of an issue for younger children, but could be a huge issue for teenagers, who might experience humiliation and an acute lack of self-confidence as a result of Long Covid. Being a teenager is hard enough without being effectively exiled and so compromised in terms of health. Adults with Long Covid will know there's only so much happening in your life that you can talk about with people who are well, given that you might not be able to participate in your usual activities or hobbies or even exercise or work. This can have a huge impact on your identity and could mean that you simply don't have as much to talk about as you used to. Teenagers might experience similar problems. In addition, maintaining conversations can be exhausting when you have Long Covid, and teenagers might be less likely to understand this and so assume that their peers with Long Covid are being rude if they are struggling to talk or listen. Long Covid Kids has received reports of increased bullying and isolation among children with Long Covid as a result.

PSYCHOLOGY

The teenage years are an emotional and psychological rollercoaster at the best of times. Being a teenager during a global pandemic is even worse. Being a teenager in a pandemic with a long-term condition that is barely understood and that seemingly no one can help with is another level of horrendous. On top of that, there's the constant threat of another wave, which could exacerbate everything even more.

There are additional factors to consider associated with Long Covid that are specific to teens. At a time when eating disorders are becoming more common, a Long Covid diagnosis that causes loss of normal taste or disgust at the taste of common foods could increase the risk of a segue into eating disorders.

Sammie from Long Covid Kids describes how children and teenagers with Long Covid might feel like they have a personal responsibility to protect their peers and families from developing the condition. The children want people to know about Long Covid, because they don't want others to end up as ill as they are. These kids feel the burden not just for themselves, but for their siblings, their parents and their teachers. They feel it for everybody, because they know what it's like to live with this condition.

Then there are the difficulties caused by being disbelieved. Imagine you're ten years old and you've always been taught to tell the truth and not to keep secrets, or to tell an adult if you have a problem. Imagine then telling the truth about how you feel and being met with disbelief (to an even greater extent than adult long haulers are), told that your symptoms are 'in your head' or caused by anxiety, or that you 'just need to try harder'. Hopes might get raised by the prospect of a medical appointment at which you will finally be listened to, treated and perhaps even cured. But the reality is that the doctors almost always tell children with Long Covid that there's nothing they can do. They advise children that they just need to get on and find a new way of living. Long Covid Kids have received reports of a lot of children being told they have a functional neurological disorder, a vague catch-all diagnosis which to all intents and purposes seems like an opportunity to stop offering care. Sammie reports that most parents and children who take their kids to see a GP about Long Covid report unsatisfactory outcomes.

So, while the symptoms of Long Covid are hugely distressing in themselves, the true measure of the impact of the condition on children in the long term may well be the psychological trauma they endure as a result.

Why is research on children with Long Covid so hard?
Research involving children is much more challenging than that in adults because of the ethics approval involved. Fundamentally, ethics committees don't like researchers going to sick children and taking blood for research (as opposed to blood tests for treatment or diagnostic purposes). That's also most likely why we know less about paediatric and adolescent immunity – because it's much harder to get proposals that involve taking blood from thousands of ten-year-olds past ethics committees.

Despite the fact that academics and researchers have spent the whole of the pandemic on fast-forward, for at least half of that time we were being told that we couldn't or shouldn't study children, because Covid wasn't a thing in children. That means there's been far less chance to study the disease in children than in adults. However, I'm very pleased that at Imperial College London we're now working more and more with some of the paediatric Long Covid groups, with paediatricians like Dr Nathalie MacDermott and Dr Liz Whittaker, to try to get to the bottom of what's going on in children with Long Covid. Some of the most important work that paediatricians and immunologists are doing is simply saying that paediatric Long Covid exists and we need to do something about it.

Challenges for parents of children with Long Covid

Here are just some of the challenges that parents with children who have Long Covid are facing:

- lack of access to flexible learning, which affects parents' ability to work
- transportation challenges in getting children whose mobility and energy are impacted to and from school
- reduced income because of having to take time off work
- unsupportive employers
- extra outgoings because of treatment costs, such as prescriptions
- mental and physical symptoms, driven by a sense of guilt and hopelessness
- inability to trust judgement, particularly when close support networks (e.g. partners, grandparents) are not supportive
- concerns about maintaining normality for siblings in a distressing situation in which the affected child might need more attention
- domestic abuse – both emotional and physical – in relationships that previously didn't feature it has been

    reported to Long Covid Kids (directed at both the parent and the affected child)

- poor knowledge and awareness in primary healthcare settings, including inaccurate diagnoses, gaslighting, minimisation of symptoms or experiences, lack of treatment options and long waiting times
- inability to relax or socialise, either because of the time pressures of caring for an ill child or concerns about exposing the family to another Covid infection
- feelings of resentment such that the parent feels like the child's health situation is holding them back
- feelings of isolation due to lack of knowledge or awareness in social circles and a lack of validation in the absence of a clear clinical definition of Long Covid.

Now, imagine that this parent also has Long Covid themselves ...

How do children's immune systems differ from those of adults? How has the narrative around children and Covid changed?

Like other systems in the body, the cells of the immune system change across the life course. Throughout development, T cells mature in the thymus (a gland between the lungs in which white blood cells mature) and then move out into the surrounding blood and lymphoid organs (such as the bone marrow, spleen and lymph nodes). But as we age, the thymus shrinks and T cells become more exhausted (as discussed in chapter 2). Meanwhile our immune memory builds throughout childhood as we are exposed to bacteria, viruses and vaccines.

During the pandemic, there have been attempts to explain why children seem to have a different susceptibility to Covid. One hypothesis was that children are more exposed to common cold viruses and therefore have more residual cross-reactive immunity to Covid as a result. However, there still isn't a satisfactory answer.

We do know that the experience of Covid in children and adolescents has been different to that of adults. It has also been different in each of the waves that we've had. In the first wave, and to a degree with the Alpha variant in general, politicians felt secure in saying that Covid wasn't a disease of children. That changed with the Beta variant, when it became apparent that children were getting infected. As Delta and Omicron arrived, the whole demographic of infection changed and the pandemic became supported by a network of infections among children in schools around the world. Even if a lower proportion of children than adults were getting severely infected or persistently affected, at a time of such high prevalence, this in the end becomes a large absolute number.

That's the point we're at now: Covid is an infection for which we ought to think about children a lot. We're in the early days of figuring out what Long Covid looks like in children, but we know that a lot of children have it. We know that it looks similar – but not identical – to the condition in adults. But it's going to take research to unpack this further, and for the reasons I mentioned in the last boxout, this may not happen quickly.

What rates of recovery can we expect in children?

If you ask the parents of children who've had Long Covid since the first wave how 'recovered' they'd estimate their child to be, they would probably give you a different answer from the child's healthcare providers. Healthcare providers often deem a patient to be recovered if they no longer need to see them. However, the reality is that patients (or their parents) often feel like healthcare professions have nothing to offer them in terms of treatment, and that it is pointless and draining to attend appointments only to have their hopes of help dashed. So, the patients end the relationship with the healthcare profession and both sides take a different perspective on why that patient is no longer coming in for care.

I asked Sammie from Long Covid Kids about the rates of recovery that she's seeing among members of her group. The children who were infected during the first wave in March 2020 and subsequently developed Long Covid have generally been improving, and may now be at something like 60 to 80% of their pre-Covid health two years on. However, it's debatable whether that can be described as 'recovery', because even if they are 60 to 80% recovered there are still many things that these children cannot do. Many are living a modified and adapted lifestyle and are still not back to their normal activities or an active life.

How many children in the group are making complete recoveries? Not many, sadly, although it's possible that those who have recovered leave the group and don't return to let others know about it. Sammie told me that she'd tried to post a positive 'giving people hope' message on the Long Covid Kids group, saying that she'd felt like she'd been through the five stages of grief and come out the other side, through anger and frustration to a place of acceptance. She'd wanted to show other parents who were in a bad place that you can come through it. Many people were genuinely pleased – the Long Covid Kids group is like a family – but few could relate. They were still angry and frustrated because life was simply so difficult when caring for a child (or children) with Long Covid. The reality is really, really hard. And rather than try to put a positive spin on it in this book, I want to call out that reality and let you, the reader, know that if you're feeling this way you're not alone. It really is that difficult, and it's OK to feel angry and frustrated about the monumental impact that Long Covid has on everyone's lives. We'll talk more about the impact on mental health in chapter 7.

What does recovery from other post-viral conditions look like in children?

The subset of patients in the big glandular fever studies who aren't back to normal one or two years later is actually quite small. Interestingly, the immune system and EBV's behaviour tend to return to normal around the same time – i.e. the virus is put back in its box and returns to being latent at the same time as T-cell concentrations fall to normal levels. However, we're not seeing the same rates of recovery in children or adolescents with Long Covid, which suggests that there's something more to the disease mechanism in this case.

Advice for parents

Perhaps the most pertinent question for concerned parents is about what can they actually do to help get their child's life back to normal. If we start at the point of catching Covid, the most important thing to reduce the risk of developing Long Covid is the same in adults and children. Based on both Long Covid Kids' observations and my own data from the adult community, it seems safe to say that *convalescence* is of the utmost importance. This doesn't necessarily mean sitting or lying completely still at all times. Rather, the advice is to think very carefully about activities that cause significant exertion. So, for some children, gentle table tennis might be OK, but the high rates of sprinting, stopping and impact in games like football, hockey or rugby might not be.

How long should this convalescence last? Sammie recommends at least two to three months if they're still experiencing symptoms after their acute infection. It's obviously hard to get children to stay still, and they're going to want to join in with whatever their friends are doing, but if they still have symptoms two or three weeks after initial infection (including a decrease in energy), this is the point when an intervention could make a massive difference. It's a hard thing to ask of a parent, but don't just take my word for it. There are now 10,000 families in the Long Covid Kids group, and Sammie believes that over-exertion in the early weeks and months after infection could have played a part in triggering the onset of the condition in most cases. This is borne out by my data on a survey of adult long haulers who had either mild or asymptomatic acute infections. Over half of them could identify overexertion as being the trigger for the onset of Long Covid, up to three months after their acute infection.[11] One useful resource (see page 283) is the 'Cautious Tortoise', an easy-to-follow flow chart that helps parents and guardians navigate the early steps of their child's recovery.

It's hard to handle illness in younger children, especially as you're never quite sure if they're as ill as they are saying they are (or as ill as they are acting). But if you have any suspicions that your child has post-Covid symptoms, it's incredibly important to believe them when they say they're in pain or suffering but aren't perhaps quite able to describe it. The best thing you can do for your child is to be a solid place of emotional support, and that starts with your child knowing they can trust you with their feelings and not be disbelieved. If you've experienced Long Covid as an adult, you'll know how hard it is to deal with people who minimise or deny your experience. It's even harder for young people dealing with the condition, as they may not have the language to describe what they're going through.

It's possible that you will face opposition from primary healthcare providers when you seek help and treatment for your child. Persistence here is key. It's frustrating that you should need to fight so hard for your child's care, but in the world of Long Covid it's an all-too-common unfortunate reality. It is possible to receive care and referrals to specialists, but you may need to keep going back to make your GP listen. If that fails, consider changing your GP. As ever, in an overstretched and under-resourced NHS, it can never do any harm to be a consumer who is always polite, yet informed and persistent!

These are the three top pieces of advice suggested by Long Covid Kids, but I still had questions for Sammie, so this Q&A includes a response from her as well as from Danny.

GEZ: What do you wish you'd known from the start?

SAMMIE: I wish I'd known that you can't just push through, that you have to rest. Simply wishing yourself well, wishing that you can please others by trying to be well, doesn't work. The other thing for parents who themselves have Long Covid is to be kind to yourself. Because you can't pour from an empty cup.

GEZ: Danny, can you tell me what help was available from medical communities for kids and adolescents who presented with long forms of viral conditions before Covid?

DANNY: There hasn't been any treatment established for glandular fever other than rest, essentially. The need for an EBV vaccine is clear and one is now being trialled, but obviously that doesn't help people who are ill now. As things stand, there's virtually nothing on the shelf to offer until, as in adult Long Covid, we can figure out what is actually happening in the condition, Ganciclovir is occasionally used in very extreme examples of EBV infection in immunocompromised people.

GEZ: How important do you think it is to answer the question: 'What's going on with Long Covid in kids?'

DANNY: The whole of the Covid experience in the end, like so many things nowadays, has become a polarised dispute. It's almost a political dispute between the laissez-faire libertarians who claim that Covid is just another infection and that we should simply get on with things and the people who are perceived as authoritarian pro-lockdowners or fearmongers. I try to be quite a calm, sanguine person most of the time, but I've spent the past several months hearing and reading about every school in the country with a fifth or a quarter of their kids missing at any given time, based on ONS data at the peak of the first Omicron wave. And if even only 1% of these children are going to have extreme persistent consequences that blight their childhood, their education and their family, then what's happening to them is criminal. I find it very hard to be calm about that.

Summary

Given that the scale and severity of Long Covid in children and adolescents has barely registered in print and broadcast media and that medical research into the condition lags interminably, it's very easy to feel alone if you're the parent of a child who has Long Covid. However, an increasing number of resources for children and young people are available, including advice on schooling, socialising and general support for parents. The latest resources are signposted at the end of the book (page 281). For now, though, we move onto perhaps the biggest question of all: what's causing Long Covid?

CHAPTER 4: What Causes Long Covid?

What's causing Long Covid? To describe this as a million-dollar question would be to substantially undervalue it. The National Institute for Health and Care Research (NIHR) in the UK has so far allocated two tranches of £20 million each to research funding for the condition, while the US National Institutes of Health (NIH) have allocated $1.2 billion to researching the long-term consequences of Covid in the 'RECOVER Trial'. But for now the potential causes of Long Covid remain unclear.

Since early in the pandemic five potential causes of the illness have been suggested:

- immune system dysregulation
- autoimmunity
- viral debris
- viral persistence
- end-organ damage caused by the virus.

More recently, we have also seen evidence that latent viruses in the body can be reactivated by SARS-CoV-2. It has been suggested that the virus may also disrupt the body's microbiome – that is the community of microbes that live in and on our bodies.[1] So, we can add two more to the hotlist:

- reactivated viruses
- disrupted microbiome.

Of course, there may be more potential causes that have yet to be identified, but there is an excellent chance that what's causing Long Covid is going to associated with one or more of these categories.

One note on this chapter: by necessity, there will be a lot of technical detail. Long Covid is complex, and it's impossible to describe what's going on without getting down into the weeds of the process.

However, Danny and I will do our best to make it as accessible as possible for all readers, no matter your existing knowledge base.

How do we simplify the picture of what's causing Long Covid?

There are different perspectives on this, but fundamentally it's a complex picture. There are now at least 50 million people on Earth who are living with the long-term consequences of a new viral infection, and they all look different. Some people have relapsing and remitting symptoms that come and go, whereas others have more stable disease; some have nervous system symptoms, others have gut symptoms and yet more have cardiac or respiratory symptoms. Not just that, but some people experience one set of symptoms one year and then another set the next year. We are all different, so people with Long Covid might not all be affected by precisely the same disease process. Why should the disease necessarily be functioning in the same way in a child with rashes on their feet and an elderly man with brain fog? What would be the common mechanism between them? And if you look at the literature, you could probably find enough mechanisms to differentially explain lots of different symptoms.

On the other hand, you could also look at my favourite Long Covid comparison, lupus – a disease that looks infinitely varied and variable, yet comes from making autoimmune antibodies against your DNA. From that single cause ensue problems in the blood vessels, kidneys, lungs and central nervous system. So, in the context of Long Covid, I'm trying to consider both possibilities: that there may be multiple disease mechanisms in play or that there could be one main cause that is manifesting in lots of different ways.

How do these causes end up creating the symptoms we experience? Well, each has the potential to wreak havoc in a number of different body systems and to create numerous pathologies (such as inappropriate blood clotting or poor cell function), each of which might result in a number of consequential symptoms. We currently have seven potential causes, a (conservative) minimum of twelve pathologies, and up to 203 symptoms associated with Long Covid.

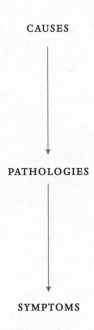

CAUSES

PATHOLOGIES

SYMPTOMS

The pathologies

So, what are these pathologies? Here's a list of 'what's going wrong' in long haulers according to an ever-increasing number of published papers (although it should be noted that we are still so early in our research into the condition that not all these findings have had a chance to be replicated across multiple studies):

- poor oxygen transfer to peripheral blood vessels
- cerebral hypoperfusion (poor blood flow to the brain)
- dysfunctional metabolism (i.e. disrupted and less effective body chemistry)

- dysfunctional mitochondria (known as the 'powerhouses' of the cell because of their role in creating energy) and RNA alterations (RNA works with DNA to produce proteins)
- microclotting, hypoperfusion (reduced blood flow) and rogue production of fibrin (a protein important in blood clotting)
- endotheliitis (inflammation of the lining of blood vessels)
- disrupted immune subsets, leading to abnormal inflammatory function
- mast cell activation syndrome (MCAS; a subset of immune dysfunction leading to distinctive patterns of inflammation and allergy previously discussed in chapter 1)
- autoimmunity of varying types, including antiphospholipid antibodies (a specific type of autoantibody that can lead to blood clots), as well as autoantibodies affecting the skin, central nervous system and heart
- small fibre neuropathy (in which damage to peripheral nerves creates pain or tingling)
- overactive microglia (immune cells in the central nervous system) and brain inflammation.

And this is even before we get to the damage that is caused by SARS-CoV-2 itself, including:

- lung damage
- heart inflammation
- liver damage
- kidney damage
- neuroinflammation and nerve damage (including to the vagus nerve)
- central nervous system pathology, including olfactory system damage.

These lists are just what we know about at the moment, and as such are far from exclusive.

This chapter and the next chapter are linked. Here we will address the hypothetical causes of Long Covid, interrogating each of them in turn. In the next chapter, we will move on to discuss the pathologies. At the end of chapter 5, we will reach the best conclusion we can about what might be causing Long Covid.

How might a dysregulated immune response be responsible for Long Covid?

Without banging too much on the same drum, a good example of a viral comparison to Long Covid is EBV. If you've been infected with a virus, it might affect your immune system in such a profound way that some aspects of your immune regulation might not be the same for a long time to come.

We've all seen those shots in films and TV shows where they zoom in from outer space, on to a country, then a town, then a street, then a house, etc. If we were to do the same thing with blood, you'd first see a red liquid, then you'd zoom in to see the separate plasma, red blood cells, platelets and white blood cells. Zooming in on your white blood cells, you'd see that they come in different shapes and sizes, and that quite a lot of them look like footballs and have large nuclei (the part of cells where DNA is stored): these cells are known as lymphocytes. When I was a student, we understood that there were two types of lymphocytes: T cells (which killed tumours and viruses) and B cells (which made antibodies). Now that we have the technology to zoom in even closer and examine the surface of these cells and their different proteins, we know that there are many thousands of gradations within the two, as well as other categories like natural killer cells and innate lymphoid cells.

The immune system, then, is made up of tens of thousands of incredibly specialist subsets that all evolved for subtly different functions that are essential to your survival. Recently published data suggests that particular subsets are perturbed in people who have Long Covid symptoms.[2] That finding seems resonant with diseases like glandular fever, because after you're infected with EBV, your body produces a lot of specific T cells called CD8 cells to try to control the infection (CD8 T cells kill cells that have been invaded by viruses and bacteria). These CD8 T cells, focused on finding cells affected by EBV, take over a sizeable part of your whole CD8 T-cell repertoire, which seems to be correlated with persistent symptoms. How? Well, if you jump from a baseline of just 0.05% of your CD8 T cells patrolling for viruses to 40% of your CD8 T cells looking for EBV, then there are going to be some knock-on effects.

These T cells are cytotoxic (harmful to cells) and they produce cytokines (inflammatory proteins involved in the immune response). Patients with glandular fever and patients with Long Covid have higher levels of these cytotoxic T cells in their blood than do healthy people.[3] Thus, the role of disrupted immune subsets and over-production of killer T cells in Long Covid is certainly worthy of further investigation, but the answers aren't clear yet.

Another possible consequence of much of your immune response being dominated by a specific type of T cell is that your immune system might be less effective at responding to other infections. During the early days of my Long Covid journey in 2020, I struggled with repeated skin infections, both bacterial and fungal (it wasn't pretty), despite never having experienced these sorts of problems pre-Covid.

The immune dysregulation explanation might also make sense to the many long haulers who experience inflammatory symptoms – be they respiratory, dermatological or gastrointestinal in nature. According to anecdotal evidence in the online support groups, anti-inflammatory diets might help to manage symptoms (see chapter 9 for further discussion of one particular anti-inflammatory diet).

We've addressed what autoimmunity is in the previous chapters, but now let's take a closer look at how it might be driving Long Covid symptoms.

How might autoimmunity be responsible for Long Covid?

As a card-carrying autoimmunity aficionado for most of my career, I ought to be careful to avoid seeming like a child with a hammer who sees everything as a nail. I may be biased towards looking for autoimmune responses everywhere, but in Long Covid there are actually some pretty strong reasons to have such a focus.

As we discussed in the previous chapter, one of the challenges that the immune system faces is how to tell the difference between the good things you want in your body and the bad things you don't. Your white blood cells have the ability to randomly rearrange amino acids (the building blocks of proteins) to produce billions of different receptors on their surface which can detect every possible protein shape in the world (and thus protect from any possible pathogen). The issue is that if they can do that, these cells can also produce receptors that can recognise your retina, for example, which isn't ideal. So, your body needs to figure out how to get rid of the cells and receptors that recognise your retina while keeping the ones that are going to recognise, say, Ebola virus. In most of us, the body can do this extremely well most of the time – that is to say that most of us, most of the time, do not have autoimmune diseases.

What's essential here is what is known as self-tolerance (discussed in chapter 2), which works in two ways. One is that the thymus (the lymphoid organ that sits between your lungs) acts as mission control for editing that white blood cell repertoire

---

and turning off everything in the cells that recognises parts of your own body. Then there's a process called peripheral tolerance, whereby any autoimmune cells that escape by mistake from this thymus control are regulated, controlled and ultimately turned off. Immunologists get very excited about things called regulatory T cells, which patrol the body and dampen down any rogue autoimmune cells to prevent autoimmune reactions. In a nutshell that's autoimmunity.

There are many different autoimmune diseases, including common ones like rheumatoid arthritis, which probably affects about 1% of the total population, less common ones like thyroiditis and lupus, and rare conditions like Sjögren's syndrome or myasthenia gravis.

In most cases, it's hard to specifically link an autoimmune disease to an infectious disease – they just happen. A prototypic example of autoimmunity following an infection is reactive arthritis, an autoimmune disease usually precipitated by a defined bout of a bacterial infection (such as salmonella), followed a few weeks later by a classic set of arthritis-like symptoms. We know that infections can mangle that immune repertoire and cause autoimmunity. One potential explanation is molecular mimicry, which is the idea that something on the surface of the invading bacterial cells resembles something in your joints, which confuses your immune system and results in an autoimmune response. This hypothesis is doing the rounds at the moment as an explanation for how Epstein-Barr virus might be associated with MS.

One of the factors that supports the role of autoimmunity in Long Covid is the preponderance of long haulers who report autoimmune issues in their immediate families. Taken with the findings discussed in chapter 2, it's possible that there's a genetic autoimmune component to the equation. This is still anecdotal and awaits larger studies.

Anecdotally, some long haulers experience temporary relief when they take corticosteroids (such as prednisolone, which is commonly prescribed for a variety of issues – in my case inflammatory skin problems). Given that corticosteroids act as immunosuppressants, this is perhaps not surprising: the steroids could be helping to calm down either an inappropriately overactive immune response or a degree of autoimmunity. However, steroids should not be taken for long periods of time because they are associated with lots of damaging side effects. Furthermore, they won't necessarily do anything to resolve the underlying trigger for the (auto)immune problems either.

More research is definitely required – and fortunately Danny is running a large project at Imperial College London that will hopefully shine some more light on this.

Now, let's turn our spotlight on the next potential culprit in our identity parade: reactivated viruses.

What role might reactivated latent viruses play in Long Covid?

Researchers like to point to EBV, which, as we know by now, is a herpesvirus. The next most ubiquitous, troublesome member of that family is another virus that many of us carry: cytomegalovirus. EBV and cytomegalovirus can both linger latently in your body for your whole life, especially in your lymphocytes, and they can sometimes cause trouble by reactivating. These two viruses play a big role in interactions with the human immune system, precisely because they're around in so many of us for life and stimulate large populations of immune cells.

In chapter 2 we discussed a paper published in the journal *Cell* in which researchers did extensive molecular immunological analyses in people with persistent Long Covid symptoms and compared the findings with those who didn't have persistent symptoms.[4] They tracked people from acute infection to persistent symptoms, and one of the things they found was statistically significant evidence of EBV reactivation at the time of acute infection. For now, we haven't a clue what that actually *means* in practice, and it raises a lot of follow-on questions, but I think it's an important finding.

If we dig down, the larger question becomes 'Could Long Covid be a specialist subset of consequences due to EBV reactivation?' I wouldn't have an ideological problem with that explanation – it's a possibility, and in science we always have to be open to possibilities. So how could EBV cause Long Covid symptoms? Well, it's a virus that has probably been piggybacking in your B cells (whose job is normally to produce antibodies) and in the cells in your throat for a number of years. It has a very complex life cycle, and can be more or less invisible and cause no bother or can reactivate all of its armoury, come out all guns blazing and cause all sorts of terrible problems. It also has the ability to transform B cells to make them cancerous, which results in diseases like Burkitt's lymphoma and nasopharyngeal carcinoma.

Usually, our patrolling CD8 T cells do a good job of keeping EBV in check, but it's a fine balance. It doesn't seem outlandish to me to believe that a new virus could completely rock that equilibrium, and just through that mechanism alone do some serious damage.

My personal experience is somewhat in alignment with the idea of reactivated EBV forming some part of the Long Covid jigsaw puzzle. I got glandular fever at age twenty-one during my final year of university. I was in dire straits for a year – suddenly all the things that should have been part of my uni experience (partying, sports, drinking, studying) were no longer possible. I saw three different GPs, each of whom did some blood tests and told me I was fine. I very much knew I wasn't, though. I felt – and looked – terrible. One of the signatures of that time was something I called a 'grizzled' feeling in my throat and chest, a sensation that I'd not had at any previous point in my life. After twelve months, I eventually recovered. I didn't experience that grizzled feeling again until twenty-one years later, a few weeks into my initial Covid infection.

That grizzled feeling prompted me to make my first YouTube film back in April 2020, which looked at the science that might link Covid to protracted post-viral symptoms. Danny's discussion of how EBV can flare up in the throat may well have been what I was experiencing a few weeks into Covid. The grizzled feeling soon went away (although Long Covid sadly didn't), and I didn't get that grizzled feeling again until – yep, you guessed it – I caught Omicron two years later.

In my personal experience, my post-EBV symptoms and Long Covid did not feel the same. Long Covid has been far more severe, has had far more kaleidoscopic symptoms and overall has been far more debilitating. To date, it has also lasted more than twice as long as my post-EBV symptoms.

Based on my own experiences, I personally don't think that Long Covid is driven *exclusively* by EBV, although reactivation of EBV and other latent viruses may certainly be adding some spice to the unpalatable Long Covid dinner we've all been served up.

How might viral debris be responsible for Long Covid?
Let's start by explaining what viral debris actually is. When SARS-CoV-2 gets up your nose, it attaches to receptors on the outside of cells, then burrows its way inside and hijacks the machinery of the cell to start producing copies of itself. These copies then go on to do the same thing to other cells in turn.

When the virus is hiding inside the cell, acting as a kind of parasite, you need some pretty fancy ways of dealing with it, including antibodies.

Antibodies are actually just a small part of the story, though, because in order for them to work they need to be present at the very first moments to stop the virus ever getting into cells. The next line of defence is the primitive detection method inside every cell that says, 'Hey, we've recognised some nucleic acid sequences that shouldn't be here. Let's detonate all forces and get rid of them.' These are what we call innate defence mechanisms (technically, interferons). They kick off in the cell the second they see a virus and try to expunge it.

If these defence mechanisms don't work, then you have a replicating virus. Part of the SARS-CoV-2 life cycle involves expressing proteins, such as the spike protein (which is famously one of the distinguishing features of SARS-CoV-2) and nucleocapsid (which some lateral flow tests detect the presence of). As soon as those proteins start to appear on human cell surfaces, patrolling T cells recognise them and activate. The only way these T cells can defend our body against the virus is by killing the infected cell. Once they've killed the cell, everything that was in that cell – including all the bits of virus – are let loose, and then you have viral debris floating around that is then mopped up by other white blood cells.

Once the white blood cells have collected the debris, they break it down. But this isn't a passive process – it's also inflammatory. These cells are also saying, 'Hey, there's something here that shouldn't be, let's get activated.' So all of this is turning on immunity, so to speak.

Now, if we go back to early 2020, the scientific thinking was that coronaviruses didn't hang around in the body or have any kind of long-term impact. To be honest, I would have sworn to that, quite far on through the pandemic. But I know that a lot of people with Long Covid felt that there must be some other answer. They felt like they'd never quite cleared the virus and never quite come out of the acute phase. I was completely agnostic on that, but did think, *That is not really how coronaviruses behave.* Then a few things emerged that started to cause some niggling doubts.

We were plotting the trajectory of acute infections in real-time in a way that we'd never really done before for an infectious disease. In the process, we were seeing that there were some people for whom it clearly took an awfully long time to get a negative result on a PCR test. Then a group of researchers in China published a very respectable letter in *The Lancet Gastroenterology & Hepatology* showing that PCR tests done on stool samples could be positive months after initial infection with SARS-CoV-2.[5] The question then became, 'Does a positive PCR result indicate the presence of live virus or of viral debris?' This is the point when I started to realise that we might need to reconsider our decades-old thinking about coronaviruses.

The story now moves to a superb research group in New York, who had previously been prominent in HIV research before turning their hands to Covid.[6] They published a really well-argued paper in *Nature* in which they essentially said, 'There's something weird going on here because, although immune and antibody responses normally wane over time, instead there are some people in whom they're actually going up. The immune system is behaving as if there's an internal driver repeatedly stimulating it.' This was such a neatly argued paper. The cherry on top was that they did gut biopsies on some of these people and detected SARS-CoV-2 or SARS-CoV-2 proteins in the gut. The researchers were unable to establish conclusively whether the virus they detected was live and capable of replication, however. Another interesting iteration of this viral persistence theme comes from a leading 'biomarker discovery' team at Harvard University, who recently showed (in a yet-to-be-peer-reviewed preprint) that they could detect the spike antigen from the virus in 60% of people with Long Covid, but not in people who had a full recovery.[7]

So, at this stage I think that viral debris is a real possibility. I haven't seen the datasets to know how common it is, but it can't be so rare because it's been detected relatively easily in some patients. I don't think viral debris alone could possibly explain all or most cases of Long Covid. There are real avenues here for treatment. These are people you could treat with monoclonal antibodies (artificially manufactured antibodies that are injected into the body), antivirals or vaccination and expect to get immediately better. And that's such an achievable experiment. The problem for the moment, though, is to square the circle by proving that persistent viral stimulation is really correlated with, and causal in, Long Covid.

In one paper well known to the Long Covid community, researchers found viral debris in monocytes (the body's 'rubbish collectors') more than a year after infection.[8] How long viral debris normally stays in the body after being broken down remains unknown, but it seems unlikely that we should have debris still hanging around for more than a year. Rather more likely is the possibility that there's a reservoir of live virus still somewhere in the body, resulting in fresh debris on an ongoing basis.

As time has gone on, more and more evidence has been published suggesting the persistence of live virus: in the lung tissues of macaques,[9] the brains of hamsters,[10] and the breast tissue[11] and even brains[12] of humans (this last study looked at autopsy results, as taking brain biopsies from living people is rather difficult). Another study found that 12.7% of participants continued to shed SARS-CoV-2 RNA in their faeces four months after diagnosis and 3.8% were still shedding seven months after the initial infection.[13] Another study detected the presence of viral RNA in the gut mucosa (the lining of the intestine) in thirty-two of forty-six patients with inflammatory bowel disease an average of 219 days after initial infection, whose stool samples *did not* test positive for SARS-CoV-2.[14] Other individual cases in which the virus persists in the gut have been reported, but larger studies have not yet been done – perhaps due to the difficulties associated with obtaining biopsies.[15, 16]

Although live virus has not been detected in blood samples provided by long haulers, in one study researchers found that 45% of their sample of patients with persistent symptoms at least four weeks after initial infection had detectable viral RNA (i.e. debris) in their blood plasma.[17]

So, while all the circumstantial evidence is pointing towards Colonel Mustard in the billiard room, we don't yet have the smoking gun to show really solve this game of Cluedo – yet. But viral persistence does make a lot of sense.

How might viral persistence be driving Long Covid?

If we assume that there is some degree of virus persisting in people's systems, we need to establish whether this is particular to long haulers, or whether everyone who has had Covid retains some virus in their system. In other words, we need to figure out if viral persistence is associated with persistent symptoms? Obviously, the persistent presence of SARS-CoV-2 would seem to make a lot of sense as a cause of Long Covid. This model gets us nearer to the EBV comparison where you've got a bruiser of a virus that hangs around in your body forever dysregulating things, rather than a common cold-like virus that somehow does something heavy duty and chronic.

Clearly there are enormous similarities between ME / CFS and Long Covid. If you look at old research papers about ME / CFS, it's almost like a foretelling of Long Covid: they describe a disease process, generally considered post-infectious, which relapses and remits and causes symptoms including fatigue, cognitive impairment, orthostatic intolerance and cardiovascular problems.

Whenever I've appeared in the media to discuss Long Covid, I've encountered a certain level of irritation, pushback and even anger from people with ME/CFS, with comments along the lines of, 'So, why is this only of interest to you now? Where were you when we needed your help so badly over past decades?' The only possible answer I could give was that medical research funding priorities are often quirky and driven by fashion and, because research is expensive, only about 10% or so of topics get funded. I also emphasise that at least we can now make up for lost time and exploit the cross-fertilisation between ME/CFS and Long Covid to the benefit of both patient groups.

The search for infectious agents has been a little different in ME/CFS. In Long Covid, we obviously already know what the initial cause is: SARS-CoV-2. In ME/CFS, by contrast, there is no consensus on a single infectious cause, although commonly proposed viruses include EBV, cytomegalovirus, human herpesviruses 6, 7 and 8 and enterovirus. All of these viruses can persist in the body to varying degrees, often lifelong.

The emphasis in ME/CFS has been on looking at evidence of viral reactivation, for example in muscle biopsies or stool samples. An outstanding recent reappraisal of post-acute infection syndromes – and ME/CFS in particular – highlighted the considerable overlap with Long Covid.[18] We are perhaps at last entering a period of synergy through study of these similar disease presentations. While neither disease is well understood, together they function almost like a Rosetta Stone for persistent disease, with the potential for illumination of both ME/CFS and Long Covid through their commonalities.

One of my favourite studies[19] that points a finger at viral persistence involved the use of sniffer dogs (not a bad idea given that dogs have previously been shown to be sniff out cancer with a high degree of accuracy[20]). The researchers took sweat samples from forty-five long haulers and 188 healthy controls, and placed the samples in special olfaction detection cones. Then they brought in the dogs, which had been trained to detect specific 'volatile organic compounds' corresponding with acute Covid infection.

The dogs successfully sniffed out that none of the 188 control participants had Covid – they were 100% accurate. By contrast, the dogs reacted to twenty-three (51%) of the forty-five samples provided by long haulers. The study's findings prompt several questions that I would love to have answers for. The dogs are more likely sniffing the body's *response* to the virus rather than the virus itself (the virus is just some RNA surrounded by various proteins – it doesn't smell). Does this mean that this biological response has simply got 'stuck on' after clearing the acute infection, or are these long haulers still producing this response to the virus because they still have *active* virus, or viral debris? Were the dogs only 51% accurate, or were they in fact 100% accurate but only half the included long haulers still had active virus or debris triggering a biological response? The Long Covid community rather cruelly jokes that these dogs are better at diagnosing the condition than most healthcare professionals. Give them a job in the NHS pronto!

One particularly exciting recent study looked at immune subsets of Long Covid patients who had been suffering for over a year. It found that they had reduced central memory T cells and increased levels of exhausted T cells (whose function is primarily antiviral). Professor Akiko Iwasaki who led the research argued that the exhausted T cells are suggestive of a chronic antigen stimulating them – that is to say, a persistent viral presence.[21]

I spoke to microbiologist and Long Covid researcher Dr Amy Proal about the possibility of viral persistence, and she detailed how it could explain what we've seen reported in Long Covid:

1. Viral persistence may dysregulate or disable the immune response in body sites such as the gut and mouth, upsetting the microbiome and barrier integrity (which would normally keep the microbes to where they are 's'pposed' to be), leading to shedding of pro-inflammatory bacterial products into blood that activate inflammatory cytokines (which would explain all the data on disrupted immune subsets).

2. Viral persistence could perpetuate an inflammatory environment, whereby the immune system is activated by a growing number of viral or microbiome pathogen proteins, leading to autoantibody production via molecular mimicry ('friendly fire', as discussed previously). At the moment this possibility is particularly speculative.

3. Viral persistence could sustain ongoing inflammation that can be sensed by the vagus nerve (especially in the gut), which can convey a pro-inflammatory signal to the brainstem in a manner that results in common dysautonomic symptoms. In addition, microglia (immune sentinels in the brain) could be activated and drive neuro-inflammation (which may also contribute to brain fog).

It does seem that when viral persistence explains so much of what we're seeing in Long Covid that we're in the realms of Occam's Razor, where the simplest solution is usually the right one. So, if there *is* virus still in our bodies, where might it be hiding (apart from in the gut)? Dr Proal has a few suggestions, starting with the lungs. As we know, the virus enters lung tissue during the acute phase, so it would be strange not to look there. The vagus nerve also innervates (sends signalling to and from) the lung, so that could explain the dysautonomia potentially triggered by tissue inflammation.

Then there's what could be considered low-hanging fruit: the appendix, haemorrhoid tissues ('cushions' of blood vessels in the rectum, where viruses like human papillomavirus can reside) and lymph nodes (where the biggest 'battles' are often fought between immune cells, antibodies and antigens). The appendix is involved with (in simple terms) 'purifying' what's in the gut, so it makes sense to check there if we think the gut is implicated in Long Covid. The real challenge is that for this type of research tissue samples are needed that are not possible to obtain from living people, so there is a need for more post-mortem research – because there's a chance that the virus could be present in the vagus nerve or brain-stem itself.

It's a scary thought, but some evidence suggests that RNA viruses can persist in the central nervous system,[22] including a case report of a person with ME/CFS who had enterovirus (a type of RNA virus that usually only causes mild disease) in their gut and in the brainstem itself.[23] Given that SARS-CoV-2 seems to infecting nerves, it is possible that it could persist in the nervous system. In an Italian autopsy study of two patients who died from acute Covid, the virus was detected in the vagus nerve and parts of the brainstem.[24]

More research on viral persistence is desperately needed, but get-ting the ethical approval and funding required to do the necessary biopsy studies is challenging. One hope is that we can come at the issue from another angle – trials of antivirals in people with Long Covid. If antivirals were shown to be effective in Long Covid, not only would we have a successful treatment for the condition, but it would also suggest that viral persistence was involved in the disease process, giving us a platform for further research. Trials of drug treatments like Paxlovid (a combination of the antivirals nirma-trelvir and ritonavir) in Long Covid are likely to happen sooner than trials attempting to find direct evidence of viral persistence.

There's one remaining villain in our Long Covid line-up: the dis-ruption of the microbiome.

How might disruption of the microbiome be responsible for Long Covid?

Let's start with some background about why in recent years clinical medicine has become so interested in microbiome re-search, especially in relation to the mechanisms underlying disease risk. It's been a given for many years that the body harbours many species of bacteria, viruses and fungi. Tradi-tionally, these were known collectively as 'commensals', and the idea was that they lived benignly in you or on you, but there was no particular assumption that there was any real interaction between you and them – they were just there and passively tolerated. Of course, this raised lots of (at the time) unanswerable questions, most prominently, 'If the immune system is all about detecting invading foreign species, how are all these species able to colonise the body for the entire human lifespan without immune attack?'

These questions remained unanswered mainly because we didn't have the technology to accurately sample all the microbial species present in and on the body. Over the past thirty years, however, molecular biology approaches have been developed that enabled identification of the species present via DNA sequencing. We have now been able to establish that microbial species are present on all mucosal surfaces (the skin, the nasal passages, the lungs, the vagina, etc.), and that perhaps thousands of different species are present, representing trillions of individual organisms. The oft-quoted figure is that the average human has ten times more bacterial cells than human cells. Put another way, we might be viewed not so much as independent human beings as taxis commandeered by bacteria to transport them around the planet.

Genetic sequencing of the human microbiome had immediate and obvious ramifications. If different people have different populations of microbial species in their bodies, perhaps this could play a role in how diseases affect people in different ways. For example, if identical twins have all the same genes yet only share development of diseases such as multiple sclerosis or type 1 diabetes around 40% of the time, could differing microbiome make-ups be one of the major, differential environmental contributions? Many disease processes have now been looked at to determine if disease susceptibility might be associated with differing communities of bacteria, viruses and fungi among the microbiome, especially in the gut. A great many correlations have been identified, including for the risk of multiple sclerosis, diabetes, arthritis and inflammatory bowel disease, as well as for outcomes after cancer immunotherapy.

A concept that emerged out of all this research was that 'dysbiosis' – i.e. a disrupted microbiome or one made up of unfavourable species – can cause wider physiological issues. Research then moved onto exploring mechanisms. The theory is that environmental and lifestyle differences produce microbiome differences, especially things like diet (high-fibre or high-fat diets and the use of sugar and sweeteners have been shown to affect the microbiome), or the extent to which your lifestyle disrupts your natural circadian rhythms in relation to those of the bacteria you're carrying.

The key physiological output of all this interaction is that your gut bacteria respond to all the food you've ingested and pour out a range of chemicals that interact with and modulate human cells. A simple example is that intake of fibre preferentially promotes the growth of microbial species that make short-chain fatty acids such as propionate, which has anti-inflammatory properties. This propionate acts on T cells that are producing inflammation and could thereby help to reduce disease. A major challenge in the field currently is how to design experiments that can really prove causality in a given disease process – i.e. how to disentangle microbiome differences to figure out whether they cause disease or whether the disease causes the microbiome difference. Some answers have emerged from complex studies in which microbial species were transferred between laboratory mice, or even from autoimmune or healthy humans to laboratory mice, to look for disease differences.[25]

It's not hard to see the massive appeal of microbiome research: if changes to the microbiome are implicated in settings from autoimmune disease to tumour immunity, then perhaps there are simple, accessible solutions – from dietary changes to probiotics and food supplements – that could reduce symptoms. This has obvious implications for those with Long Covid, although it is still early days in terms of research, some showing microbiome-disease correlates, others not. Larger studies are certainly warranted – in the case of Long Covid, for example, to establish if dysbiosis could drive pathogenic changes in immune and inflammatory cells. At the time of writing, there's media interest in a proposed Long Covid predictive test which is based on microbiome analysis of stool samples. While I'd never seek to peer review the work of others on the basis of a press release, it seems to me that a microbiome profile may well be interesting and informative, but might be unlikely to have the sensitivity and specificity needed for a clinically applicable test.

I've noted that gut microbiome sequencing has now been added to the long list of commercially available clinical tests for which long haulers are being asked to pay (often large sums). It is certainly fascinating to have your personal dataset for those trillions of bacterial passengers. My personal advice would be to hang on to your cash. The reason for this is that the useful answers have tended to come from very large studies comparing patient and control groups, making it hard to know what to make of just your own, personal data.

While gut microbiome tests are commercially available, they can only reveal a small part of the picture when it comes to the potential scope of the problem. Yes, most long haulers do seem to have unusual results when they take gut microbiome tests, but we don't yet have enough data to draw any conclusions across the group as a whole. Our understanding of the true scope of the microbiome in the body is still developing, and, like all the other hypotheses discussed in this chapter, more research is desperately needed.

Summary

My opinion is that the cause of Long Covid is unlikely to be a single factor – it may well be a combination of several of the causes discussed in this chapter, which might even interact with each other. This complexity makes the condition so hard to unpack, especially when the list of identified pathologies seems to be growing by the day. In the next chapter, we'll identify what the affected biological systems and processes are in Long Covid, and explore how they are 'going wrong' according to the published literature to date.

CHAPTER 5: *The Pathology of Long Covid*

Whatever the causes of Long Covid might be, they are driving a number of physiological processes to function less well than they do in a healthy individual. These malfunctioning physiological processes, or 'pathologies', are the topic of this chapter. A large proportion of these pathologies are related in some form to impaired vascular function rather than impaired respiratory function (i.e. they're related to your blood vessels as opposed to your lungs and breathing).

How has the thinking around the nature of Covid disease changed?

Early in the pandemic there was an assumption that Covid was a respiratory disease because complications in acute cases were respiratory in nature. Textbook examples of respiratory diseases, such as influenza, get into the respiratory tract and result in the production of excessive inflammatory cells, which negatively impact the transfer of oxygen from the lungs into the blood. At the beginning of the pandemic everybody was looking for the same process in Covid, and there were a few good papers suggesting that this was the primary mechanism of disease. However, it has transpired that that's not the whole story. SARS-CoV-2 infects cells via the ACE2 receptor, which is widespread throughout the human body. There's therefore no particular reason why the SARS-CoV-2 virus should solely attack the cells in the respiratory system.

A lot of the science that's been published in the past two years has been very piecemeal and has jumped around between

---

different effects of the virus – partly because they have been so unexpected. As a result, it's easy to rapidly degenerate into word association and picking common factors rather than doing rigorous analysis. But among the things we've discovered, there are a few pathologies that seem to be nailed on, and these include poor gas transfer, impaired vascular function and endotheliitis (inflammation of the lining of our blood vessels). These processes seem likely to be involved in Long Covid. This creates a picture of a condition much nearer to a vasculitis-type disease than a typical respiratory pneumonia. Viewing Covid as a vascular disease could potentially also bring all the other elements into play – like the autoimmune spectrum, varying autoantibodies, even microclots. However, as a scientist, I'm hesitant to state outright that Covid is a vascular not a respiratory disease because the evidence base is still lacking. We're still waiting for a big paper in *The Lancet* or the *British Medical Journal* to draw everything together.

The suggestion that Covid could be a vascular rather than respiratory illness might help us understand the wide range of effects observed in long haulers. In the previous chapter, we outlined a list of the pathologies that have been observed in people with Long Covid. We will now go through them one by one.

Oxygen extraction

Why is exercise so hard (and detrimental) to long haulers? Research has suggested that long haulers struggle to extract oxygen from their blood.[1] Under invasive cardiopulmonary exercise testing, patients with Long Covid in whom no abnormalities were detected in chest imaging, pulmonary function or resting heart function had significantly impaired oxygen extraction compared with healthy controls. The essential delivery mechanism for oxygen transfer simply wasn't working as well as it should. In a follow-up letter discussing these findings it was suggested that a microvascular or molecular abnormality might be causing the issue.[2] My personal thinking is that a number of factors may be involved – from dysfunctioning mitochondria (the part of the cell responsible for generating energy) to microclotting and inflammation of the endothelium.

Endotheliitis

The endothelium is the inner lining of the blood vessels. It has been well established that SARS-CoV-2 wreaks havoc on the endothelium, causing 'massive damage' during the acute infection.[3, 4] This damage to blood vessels can lead to tissue swelling, inflammation, activation of platelets (components of blood that are central to the clotting process) and impaired oxygen extraction from the blood (as the lining of the blood vessel is now too inflamed for the oxygen to pass through effectively), all for long periods after the acute infection.

Microclotting

When platelets get erroneously activated, they can promote an 'inflammatory hypercoagulable endotheliopathy'.[5] In layman's terms the linings of your blood vessels become inflamed, which upsets the natural balance of the blood, prompting it to clot more easily, which triggers more inflammation in the blood vessels, which triggers more clotting. Perhaps it's not surprising then that we see increased rates of thrombotic events (whereby blood clots travel round the body and cause problems including pulmonary embolisms, heart attacks and strokes) in the months and years following acute Covid infection.[6]

In one study well known to the long hauler community, researchers examined blood samples with a fluorescent microscope and saw not just huge, hyperactive platelet activity but also a proliferation of 'microclots' in blood plasma.[7] The wider scientific community has yet to reach agreement on the nature and composition of what was found, but for the purposes of this discussion we will take the paper at face value and refer to them as 'clots'. These clots were resistant to the body's normal breakdown processes (fibrinolysis) and contained various molecules that cause inflammation. While these clots weren't big enough to cause major thrombotic events, they were large enough to potentially block capillary beds (the network of tiny blood vessels in your muscles, organs and other tissues), which may reduce oxygen delivery. To date, these microclots have been found in every long hauler that has been tested by the research team, but none of the healthy controls.

This study only contained forty-seven participants (including healthy controls), though, and there are still some questions remaining. We don't know if people who recovered fully after acute Covid infection also have microclots (which may affect the relevance of the finding), and we don't know how high up the causality ladder these microclots are – i.e. are they responsible for a large number of the other pathologies and hence symptoms, or are they just a side effect of something else that's going wrong?

Microclots were one of the first obvious markers of disease discovered in Long Covid and are a hot topic in research. Larger research projects are underway and will hopefully answer some of these pressing questions.

Cerebral hypoperfusion

Cognitive dysfunction (often reductively referred to as brain fog) is often the second most common symptom reported (after fatigue) in most Long Covid surveys. It's very real and extremely debilitating. It can manifest as difficulties with processing new information (visual, written or verbal) or memory recall (particularly short term), and speech can become stuttering or slurred. Essentially, we're seeing problems with the input, sorting, recall and output of information. Different individuals find different things hard. Personally, I struggle with verbal processing, and as a result long conversations become increasingly difficult as the minutes wind on. Zoom calls are a nightmare. My visual processing and coordination are usually OK (apart from when I'm experiencing post-exertional malaise) but some people are so affected by these symptoms that they don't feel confident driving. For many long haulers cognitive dysfunction has a very significant impact on their quality of life. What might be causing it?

A number of studies have shown that blood flow in the brain is abnormal in people with Long Covid (even after 'mild' initial infections).[8, 9] It can either flow too slowly or in a dysregulated fashion. You don't need to be a rocket scientist to work out that this might cause oxygenation issues – and, without oxygen, brain cells aren't going to work properly. In one study researchers did brain scans in long haulers' brains to see what might be going on.[10] They found a decrease in brain activity in the olfactory gyrus (which controls taste and smell), the limbic regions (involved in memory and emotion regulation), the brainstem (which controls autonomic functions including breathing, heart rate and sleeping) and the cerebellum (which regulates motor skills and balance). The reduction in brain activity corresponded with increased symptoms.

So, what's causing these problems? Well, there's evidence that SARS-CoV-2 loves to attack pericytes through their ACE2 receptor. Pericytes are cells that surround blood capillaries and are involved in the regulation of blood flow in the brain, heart and kidneys. Neuroscientists at University College London showed that the virus blocks ACE2 receptor functioning on pericytes, causing capillaries in brain tissue in hamsters to constrict – which could explain this kind of blood flow issue.[11] Another study found that SARS-CoV-2 infected – and killed – endothelial cells (i.e. the cells that line the blood vessels) in human brains, thereby causing microvascular brain pathology.[12] So, the blood vessels in the brain might be *damaged*, as well as being constricted. Unfortunately, this isn't all SARS-CoV-2 can do to the brain – we'll come back to this later in the chapter.

Mitochondrial dysfunction

Given the role of mitochondria in energy production, it's not surprising that they've long been of interest in ME/CFS. And given the similarities between ME/CFS and Long Covid, mitochondrial dysfunction may also go some way to explaining the all-consuming nature of Long Covid fatigue. If your cells don't have the energy to power basic biological processes, how are they going to produce the energy necessary to enable your body to function normally?

It's still a little too early to have comprehensive data about the role of mitochondrial function in Long Covid. But one early data analysis showed that SARS-CoV-2 infection altered the transcription of forty-three small mitochondrial RNAs (which play an important role in regulating cellular metabolism and the use of oxygen).[13] This suggests that contact with the virus altered some of the genetic material of these mitochondria. We don't know yet what the consequences might be, but it seems plausible that altered mitochondria might not be able to create energy in the usual way.

Speaking of creating energy, in the field of ME/CFS, research has shown that when the mitochondria of people with ME/CFS are put under stress, generation of ATP (the fundamental unit of energy in the body) declines dramatically.[14] The science describing exactly how this happens gets pretty gnarly, but the way glucose is used by the cells is altered and the mitochondria instead turn to fatty acids for energy. Anyone who's experienced a Long Covid (or indeed ME/CFS) crash will find the idea that the body responds poorly to physiological stress (putting pressure on mitochondrial function) very familiar.

Why do many long haulers report swollen lymph nodes?
We immunologists spend our entire lives taking small tubes of blood out of people's arms and analysing them in fancy ways. Which is fine, but that's all people will let us do – they don't allow us to take their organs for some reason.

But mission control for all those fancy immune responses is actually in the lymph nodes. These are the small, spherical structures that you can feel in places like your armpit when you have an infection (this is what is meant by 'swollen glands'). Your immune system doesn't really work by T cells and B cells randomly bumping into invading species in your blood vessels – it's much more anatomically choreographed than that, involving quite fancy structures in your lymph nodes. So, if your lymph node has suddenly swollen to two or four or ten times its usual size, that's because there are two or four or ten times more cells in there than usual.

And they're not just random cells, they're cells that are there for a reason – usually they're attacking something. For example, when I talk about beautifully choreographed structures, the B cells that make antibodies have particular receptors on them for particular viruses and the T cells that attack the viruses have particular receptors on them too. That would be a pretty useless mechanism unless they could actually meet up in the same place, at the same time, and attack the same virus. The lymph node is where that's happening. So, if long haulers report persistently swollen lymph nodes, the clear implication is that the B and T cells at that site are receiving ongoing stimulation and are continuing to respond. The most obvious trigger to consider is persistent virus, though we might also need to consider possibilities such as the 'self antigens' that drive autoimmunity. Some researchers are starting to study the specificity and receptors of B and T cells in the lymph nodes by using a very final needle to remove some cells but this hasn't yet been done in Long Covid.

Dysfunctional metabolism

Metabolism, simply described, is the way our bodies manage chemical reactions in order to sustain life. Metabolism is absolutely fundamental, and includes the conversion of food to energy, muscle, fat and connective tissue, and the elimination of metabolic waste. To say metabolism is complex is to rather understate the point – it is almost unfathomably intricate, and the body often has more than one way of achieving certain tasks. What seems to be happening in people with Long Covid is that some of those metabolic pathways are being hijacked and the body has to compensate in a way that results in side effects – and, ultimately, symptoms.

At the moment the science detailing how this might happen is mostly still hypothetical: the effects on the metabolism can be measured, but it's hard to drill down to observe the mechanisms themselves, and experiments by and large haven't happened yet. However, the hypotheses are compelling.

One team have suggested that the absorption of tryptophan (an essential amino acid required for maintenance of the body's proteins, muscles, enzymes and neurotransmitters) might be compromised in Covid, which could explain many of the symptoms long haulers experience, including fatigue, headaches and cognitive dysfunction.[15]

Meanwhile, South African researchers have published an incredibly detailed paper describing the complex chain reaction that they believe occurs.[16] Metabolism at this level of detail gets extremely technical – to the degree that even doctors I know are bamboozled by it. However, I'll try my best to break it down in the simplest terms I can.

We've already talked about ATP – the principal molecule for storing and transferring energy in cells. Lots of ATP equals lots of energy to power the body's systems. To create ATP, we need something called NAD+, which, as we discussed way back in chapter 1, is a molecule that helps to catalyse chemical reactions in the body. The hypothesis is that NAD+ is depleted by Covid infection and subsequent inflammation. In order to get more, the body is forced to break down tryptophan, but as a consequence the body then ends up with insufficient tryptophan, which inadvertently increases production of inflammatory cytokines.

This has a couple of side effects. Excessive amounts of kynurenine and quinoloic acid – essentially waste products created by this metabolic workaround – accumulate, which can potentially cause autonomic issues, cognitive dysfunction, platelet activation and histamine intolerance.[17] The second side effect is a knock-on depletion of serotonin (a neurotransmitter important for control of mood, blood pressure and digestion) and melatonin (which helps to regulate the natural sleep cycle).

Overall, this hypothesis is compelling, and suggests that there may be a simple way to compensate for some of this metabolic madness – more on that in chapter 10.

MCAS

As briefly discussed in chapter 1, MCAS is a chronic, multi-system, inflammatory disorder that results from dysfunction of a type of immune cell known as the mast cell. Mast cells normally help to protect the body from pathogens and parasites.[18]

MCAS has only recently been acknowledged as a condition in its own right, and is frequently confused by medical professionals with mastocytosis (a rare condition in which an excess of mast cells gather in the body's tissues). MCAS is surprisingly common, and could affect up to 17% of the population.[19] The most common manifestations of MCAS are migraines, headaches, gastrointestinal problems (such as irritable bowel syndrome), fibromyalgia and even anxiety and depression. MCAS is also strongly related to allergy, but allergic symptoms are not a prerequisite for an MCAS diagnosis. Most people with MCAS won't realise they have it, and it simply doesn't get diagnosed very often because it wasn't covered at medical school when most doctors did their training.

MCAS has previously been linked to dysautonomia, and specifically to PoTS (see chapter 1),[20] but more recently it has been associated with Long Covid.[21] Researchers compared symptoms in people with Long Covid with those in people with MCAS – and the lists were nearly identical. So, what's going on? Mast cells could be activated in Long Covid by a number of means, including assault from SARS-CoV-2 directly, consequential cytokine activity, genetic deregulation and the development of autoantibodies that react with mast cell receptors.

Whatever is causing MCAS in Long Covid, when we look at the similarity in symptom presentation it does suggest that something *very* strange is going on in the neighbourhood. Who ya gonna call?

Inflammation

Inflammation is a rather general, over-arching term to describe an endpoint of immunity that favours activation and accumulation of white blood cells – mobilising the troops. As such, you could categorise the many chemicals made within the immune response (cytokines and chemokines) as either 'pro-inflammatory' – enhancing this process – or 'anti-inflammatory' – down-regulating this process. Research has suggested that inflammation is a key driver of Long Covid neurological symptoms.[22] In addition to producing a wide range of pro-inflammatory cytokines, inflammation can lead to over-activation of microglia (immune 'sentinels' in the central nervous system that can signal and attract other immune cells to attack pathogens) and astrocytes (cells that support neurons), which could be responsible for a wide range of neurological symptoms.

Dr Bruce Patterson and his team in the USA used inflammatory markers in the blood to determine a 'long hauler score', which is essentially a pattern of cytokine profiles that seem to be specific to Long Covid patients.[23] In another paper, this group detailed how viral RNA fragments were discovered in non-classic monocytes (the 'rubbish collectors' of the immune system) and theorised that these monocytes could drive the inflammation that causes the symptoms of Long Covid.[24] From my perspective, the question is 'Where in the causality chain are these cytokines?' Are they at the top driving the symptoms, or are they just a consequence of other pathologies – essentially a side effect?

Antiphospholipid antibodies

One of the hot areas for investigation in autoimmunity in Long Covid is antiphospholipid antibodies. Antiphospholipid syndrome, also known as Hughes syndrome, is a disorder of the immune system that causes an increased risk of blood clots, due to antibodies attacking proteins that are attached to fat molecules called phospholipids (hence the name). It has been reported that antiphospholipid syndrome can be brought on by acute Covid infection, and there is a suggestion that increased antiphospholipid antibodies may be a factor in Long Covid too.[25-27] Outside of Covid, antiphospholipid syndrome normally affects women more than men, usually across early-middle age. Sound familiar?

Which autoantibodies are suspected to play a role in Long Covid?

As we've seen in chapter 2, there's good reason to consider an overarching paradigm of autoimmunity in Long Covid, not least because aspects of Long Covid are so reminiscent of autoimmune conditions such as lupus, vasculitis, pemphigus (a disease of blistering due to autoantibodies targeting against proteins on skin cells) and antiphospholipid syndrome. Even the seemingly inexplicable cycles of relapse and remission (or flare-up and resolution) that have been seen in Long Covid are straight out of the autoimmunity playbook.

There are some autoimmune diseases in which the presence of specific autoantibodies is decisive and diagnostic – think thyroiditis or antiphospholipid syndrome. Yet there are also autoimmune diseases for which a specific causative autoantibody has not been identified, such as type 1 diabetes. Even if you can find the autoantibodies, they may just be a proxy for self-reactive T cells, which, like autoantibodies, can attack the body's own DNA or tissues.

Several studies have taken the first steps in defining which autoantibodies are detected in Long Covid. They use a range of different approaches. Some look for the relatively small panel of routine autoantibodies regularly screened for in autoimmune diseases. Others have started by targeting a specific, favoured hypothesis, such as looking for a role of antiphospholipid antibodies. Then there's the more speculative approach of screening for autoimmunity more comprehensively, to many proteins in the body. Each of these approaches shows an enhanced profile of autoimmunity in Long Covid cohorts. However, because studies have also shown that just looking at serum from anyone who had an acute Covid infection can reveal an altered and enhanced array of autoantibodies, there's a little way still to go in proving which patterns are correlated with Long Covid, and with which specific symptoms.

Research thus far has made more progress in showing that SARS-CoV-2 induces autoantibodies than in proving whether these autoantibodies are a cause of Long Covid, but the direction of travel is clear. For example, an excellent paper detailed assessment of prothrombotic autoantibodies in people who had been hospitalised during acute Covid infection.[28] Infection was associated with the appearance of several different types of antiphospholipid autoantibodies. Among other things, high levels of these autoantibodies were associated with pro-inflammatory neutrophil activation. Another team of researchers focused on autoantibodies implicated in neurological symptoms, especially PoTS. In this case, they looked specifically at people with Long Covid and showed an association with patterns of autoantibodies against a family of cell receptors called G protein-coupled receptors.[29]

Dr Yu Zuo told attendees at the American College of Rheumatology conference in 2020 that over half of Covid patients were at least transiently positive for antiphospholipid antibodies (i.e. for at least some period of time during their acute infection they had active antiphospholipid antibodies), which can activate endothelial cells, platelets and neutrophils (a type of white blood cell that helps the body fight infection), thereby promoting the formation of blood clots.[30, 31] Even if you've only been skimming this chapter, you'll have noticed there are a few ideas that keep coming up – endothelitis, platelets and clotting – and in antiphospholipid syndrome it seems all three cherries line up on the fruit machine. Unlike Long Covid, though, there are relatively straightforward tests that your GP can do for antiphospholipid syndrome, so if you think you might be at risk, it is possible to find out.

How and where do we look for autoantibodies?
There are tens of thousands of proteins expressed in the human body that could theoretically become targets for autoimmune attack, but most autoimmunity research and diagnostics since the origins of the field in the 1970s have tended to focus on around 100 key candidates. In the search for autoantibodies involved in Long Covid, some have focused on trying to establish if any of these usual candidates are implicated using standard immunological tests. Others (including my

research team) have embarked on a mission to look in an open-ended way: we figure that, even if the disease process *is* caused by one of the standard autoantibodies, our comprehensive screening approach will still pick it up.

We need to carefully design studies of autoantibodies in Long Covid, because we know that acute SARS-CoV-2 infection (especially severe infection) can induce autoantibodies, including against cytokines such as interferons (which are one of our body's first lines of defence against the virus). Thus, care is needed to ensure that studies capture only autoantibodies that are specifically implicated in causing Long Covid, rather than autoantibodies that might just be lingering in the aftermath of acute infection.

Summarising the findings of the studies published to date, there is plenty of evidence for the induction of autoantibodies as a consequence of SARS-CoV-2 infection and some studies specifically make the link to Long Covid symptoms. However, it can be hard to figure out the bigger picture when studies tend to focus on one small aspect of the process or another. Assuming that these autoantibodies do have a causal role in Long Covid that can be reliably mapped, this would raise the possibility of developing diagnostic tests for the condition. Such tests would be enormously useful in terms of ensuring access to care, disability provision and (if relevant) health insurance coverage.

Organ damage

The Long Covid pathologies outlined so far could be described as 'biological processes gone wrong', which as such just need 'putting right'. That is to say, they may be reversible. However, SARS-CoV-2 also causes physical damage to various organs, and while this damage may heal over time, the mechanism by which it results in symptoms is rather different. Making a generalisation, it's perhaps fair to say that organ damage is usually associated with people who had severe acute infections and required hospitalisation or admission to the ICU. Such patients might have different needs from those who had 'mild' acute infections but do not have (potentially severe) Long Covid. This distinction between the two groups of long haulers is important, but is not often made by clinicians or in the academic literature.

So, what kind of damage can SARS-CoV-2 do? Let's start at the top. A study compared brain samples from humans found to have Covid at the time of death and from mice infected with, and recovering from, SARS-CoV-2.[32] It showed similar neuroinflammation, microglial reactivity (the brain's immune response) and levels of chemokines in both species, all of which have been associated with impairments in cognitive function. Unfortunately for the mice, subsequent analysis revealed decreased oligodendrocytes and myelin (the building blocks of the insulating layer around nerves) in their brains several weeks after infection. In plain English, it looked like the virus destroyed part of the fabric of the brain's neural connections. Given the rest of the similarities between the mice and the humans, and without long haulers willing to have their heads opened up, we're led to assume the same is true for humans.

Another study that included 785 participants rather alarmingly showed a reduction in grey-matter thickness in the brain – and indeed in total brain size – in people who had had Covid.[33] It seems that Covid can quite literally shrink your brain.

Moving down to the lungs, in another study long haulers underwent special chest scans that used xenon gas to reveal hidden damage in the lungs.[34] While normal CT scans showed nothing untoward, the scans using xenon gas showed various abnormalities that impaired gas transfer in participants with Long Covid compared with healthy controls. No wonder this group had problems with breathlessness.

As for the heart, a huge database study published in *Nature Medicine* showed that the risk of twenty different cardiovascular diseases was substantially increased in people who'd had Covid within the previous year compared with those who hadn't.[35] The more severe the initial infection was, the higher your risk, but even among people who were not hospitalised during their acute infection the risk was still higher in all categories compared with people who didn't get Covid. While we don't quite know what the physical damage is that is increasing these risks, it seems pretty safe to say that your heart isn't the same post-Covid as it was before.

In a broad study[36] looking at a number of different organ systems in 201 patients with Long Covid, MRI scans showed impairment of the heart, lungs, pancreas, kidney, spleen and liver. Overall, 70% of the long haulers studied had impairment in at least one organ, and 29% had multi-organ impairment.

One distinction worth thinking about here is 'damage' as opposed to 'impairment'. How many of these organs were not functioning normally due to poor blood flow, oxygen perfusion or a build-up of metabolic waste, all of which could be termed impairment? While SARS-CoV-2 may wreak havoc and lead to widespread cellular infection in the acute stage, it is difficult to distinguish between damage to capillary beds and poor gas transfer due to endothelial inflammation, for example. I think I can probably speak on behalf of all long haulers when I say I'd much rather have a reversible explanation than one that describes widespread organ damage. So, before any readers get too worried that there's a 70% chance a random organ of theirs is ruined for ever, these findings should be taken with a pinch of salt until we have a better understanding of what's causing the impairment in function.

While it's clear that diverse, exciting approaches to imaging of different organs in the search for post-Covid damage have been useful, it would be premature to jump to a view that Long Covid will soon be diagnosed by scanning for damage. Some of the mechanisms of pathology under discussion simply wouldn't be visible as gross structural damage to the heart, lungs or brain. These are important qualifiers to keep on board as we enter a period in which assessments in the sphere of disability benefits or health insurance may come to rest on diagnostic 'proof' of Long Covid. We are a long way from a period when imaging of end-organ damage (or the lack of it) could or should ever be decisive in such cases.

Summary

I hope that this chapter and the last have given you a better grasp of – if nothing else – the sheer complexity of the puzzle that clinicians and researchers around the world are trying to solve. My own personal take is that we're unlikely to find that just one of the 'causes' of Long Covid discussed is responsible for all the pathologies described. I'd put money on a few different causes being implicated, potentially with one 'main' cause sitting at the top, driving the others. I personally think that viral persistence is the most likely candidate to be such a main cause, given the balance of evidence we have to date. It could explain the consequential viral debris, immune system dysregulation, autoimmunity and microbiome disruption.

The variety of symptoms and presentations and complex matrix of pathologies would all make more sense if some SARS-CoV-2 never completely went away. It is worth clarifying the fact that nasal and throat PCRs are negative in all long haulers (unless they are unlucky enough to get reinfected) and that they are not infectious – whatever and wherever this viral reservoir is, it's behaving very differently from how acute infection does. Aside from effective treatment, this is perhaps the greatest single question remaining for Long Covid research to answer.

CHAPTER 6: Gender Bias and How to Tackle It

Gender bias is not a new phenomenon – it's not an exaggeration to say it has been around for as long as society has existed. Gender bias is discrimination or prejudice based on a person's gender. It can be targeted at any gender but is most commonly experienced as a systemic bias against women and girls. Sarah Graham, author of *Rebel Bodies: A Guide to the Gender Health Gap Revolution*, argues that stereotypes form a large part of gender bias, and notes that over time there has been a shift from overt or explicit expressions of gender bias (although this does still happen) towards *unconscious* bias. This can be just as impactful and is perhaps even more difficult to tackle. An example in a medical context would be a doctor ascribing symptoms such as chest pain to anxiety in female patients, instead of considering that they could be a sign of something more serious and investigating them further. It is worth emphasising that trans and non-binary people also experience significant bias in medical settings, although there are currently very few papers published on the subject.[1]

The history of how the medical establishment has perceived and treated women is illustrative of why there are still issues today. Professor Brian Hughes describes how back in ancient Greece and Rome, people interpreted female emotions as a kind of illness caused by something going wrong in the female body. This led to the word 'hysteria', which referred to a woman's uterus being out of place. There is also a tradition in science and medicine of seeing the male form as the 'default' human body and female bodies thus as a variation or even deviation. This produces the absurd situation in which women's health is seen as a specialism even in health science terms. A few years ago, NASA couldn't even send female astronauts to space because all the space suits had been designed for men. Using the male body as standard remains endemic in medicine, and both education and research are still hampered as a result.

Women's health and safety are directly at risk because of inequality and assumptions around gender. In 2018, the American Heart Association funded a study looking at how many men and women were given CPR by passers-by or their workmates after they collapsed.[2] The results showed that half of men were given CPR, but only a third of women were. Of course, both men and women can have heart attacks in public places, but there seems to be an assumption that when men collapse, it's serious, whereas when women do it's less likely to be so.

In a Swiss study published in 2018,[3] researchers looked at patients presenting to doctors with chest pain. Men are more likely to experience heart disease than are women, but when someone of any gender presents *with chest pain* it is likely to be an indication of serious heart disease. However, in the study men were twice as likely to be referred to a cardiologist as women were. Given that you're in serious trouble if you have heart disease and don't receive specialist care, this bias is literally a life-or-death issue.

Has research into conditions that predominantly affect women historically been neglected?

This has certainly been a problem in the past, and my colleagues who research topics including the menopause, hormone replacement therapy (HRT) and menorrhagia (heavy or prolonged menstrual bleeding) inform me that it is absolutely still an issue. From my personal (and therefore non-systematic) view of the landscape, research related to conditions that could come under the pejorative old term 'women's troubles' can often find itself dismissed, although there is perhaps less down-playing or reluctance to consider, say, cervical cancer or lupus. The fact remains that, in an environment in which grant panels can't fund all research applications, fashion and peer-group pressure prevail. When grant panels are gender-skewed it becomes all too possible to tacitly sideline proposals rooted in women's health as 'minority issues'! I think that this is changing, but slowly and imperfectly. I *still* get invited by funders to sit on grant panels on which men outnumber women by a magnitude of five or even ten to one.

Chronic illness

Objectively, numerically and proportionately, women are more likely to experience autoimmune diseases than are men. Dr Tania Dempsey points out that other chronic illnesses can affect women disproportionately too, from gender-specific conditions like endometriosis to less specific problems like ME/CFS, fibromyalgia, migraines and chronic cystitis, which all have a higher prevalence in women. You would think that doctors would be aware of these conditions and the fact that they affect women more than men – and hence take women with these complaints (or indeed other chronic illness) seriously. But that isn't the experience of many women who try to get help from primary care.

I spoke to Dr Nina Muirhead (who has lived experience of ME/ CFS) and she raised the point that the ten conditions that GPs most commonly see do not include these chronic illnesses that primarily affect women. According to an article in the *British Journal of Family Medicine* in 2019,[4] GPs' most common appointments are suggested to be:

- diabetes
- chronic obstructive pulmonary disease (COPD) and asthma
- dermatological conditions
- musculoskeletal issues

- high blood pressure
- heart problems
- stroke recovery
- acute illness
- cancer and palliative care
- therapeutics and managing prescriptions.

Are chronic illnesses not on this list because they are less common than these other complaints, because patients don't seek help as frequently, or because they are not diagnosed as frequently? Whatever the answer, given how busy GPs are with these other conditions, we perhaps shouldn't be so surprised at their lack of experience and intimate knowledge of chronic conditions like ME/CFS or fibromyalgia.

Dr Muirhead says that to understand the issue of gender bias in chronic and autoimmune illness you also have to consider the history of medical education and the foundation of doctor training. Women were not allowed entry into UK medical schools until the late nineteenth century, a representation of the male-centric nature of the profession.[5]

Medical students have a huge amount to learn from an ever-expanding medical syllabus in a relatively limited amount of time. The focus is generally on what not to miss in life-or-death situations – critical signs and symptoms in heart attacks, strokes or pulmonary embolisms, for example. There's a saying in medicine that 'common things are common', which is intended to focus the mind away from obscure conditions and help doctors to diagnose the most probable causes of illness.

While chronic disease is covered in medical training, there are a number of diseases that primarily affect women that are not a major focus of the syllabus. As a result, there's now a lack of understanding across the board of various chronic diseases that a lot of women have. Fibromyalgia, for example, is far more common in women and could affect up to 5% of the population, yet it takes an average of 2.3 years and 3.7 physicians to make a diagnosis.[6] According to Endometriosis UK, it takes an average of seven to nine years to be diagnosed with the condition in the UK,[7] and PoTS also incredibly takes between five and seven years to diagnose on average,[8] despite the availability of a simple initial diagnostic test (the heart rate rising more than 30 beats per minute within ten minutes of standing up). The situation is similar internationally. Although data is patchy, there is evidence suggesting that the time for initial symptom presentation to diagnosis of endometriosis is four to seven years in Brazil[9, 10] and 4.4 years in the USA.[11]

Dr Muirhead also revealed that the picture differs throughout the UK: ME/CFS, for example, takes five years to diagnose in Manchester, but nine years in Wales, according to the results of a patient survey. Dr Muirhead argues that many medics aren't even looking to make a diagnosis in the first place – the short duration of GP appointments and the absence of specific medical training means that patients with underdiagnosed chronic conditions are being neglected by the healthcare system.

Dr Muirhead suggests that women can become very good at dealing with pain, and are often encouraged by other women to 'get on with it'. How many teenage girls are told by everyone from their mothers to their teachers or sports coaches to push through and ignore medical symptoms because 'everyone gets periods, everyone gets pain; you have to live with it because you're a woman'? As a result, many women accept and tolerate high levels of pain and do not communicate their situation to their doctor or healthcare provider. This may even be a rational decision – there is evidence to suggest that caregivers and clinicians underestimate women's pain compared to men's.[12]

How the bias persists

In her book *Doing Harm*, Maya Dusenbery argues that there is both a knowledge gap and a trust gap in terms of women's healthcare, which can lead to significant bias in care.[13] Sarah Graham points out that historically more research has been done into conditions

that mostly affect men, particularly in the past when more researchers were men. Still to this day conditions that primarily affect
women get less research funding and as a result are less well understood. Both endometriosis and ME/CFS are good examples of the
resulting knowledge gap, which manifests in the astounding
amount of time it takes for diagnosis (and then appropriate treatment) of these conditions.

The trust gap results from the persisting idea that women are on
some level more emotional or irrational than men. Their perception of their symptoms is consequentially seen as less objective or
trustworthy by health professionals. When a patient has symptoms
that cannot easily be explained, it then becomes a very easy leap to
jump to the conclusion that the patient is 'making it up'. In fact,
when presented with such medically unexplained symptoms, the
speed at which GPs and clinicians come to conclusions is alarming.

What are medically unexplained symptoms?
When interviewing candidates for medical school, one of the
most usefully discriminating questions for my tastes is, 'What
does it take to be a good doctor?' Without wishing to be mean
at the candidates' expense, I would say that the most common
responses seem to be based on predicting the answer that in-
terviewers want to hear. Common qualities that come up often are things like kindness, empathy, good listening and good
communication. While all these things are obviously important, I always think that a doctor who excels in all these areas
but doesn't know enough about medicine to actually *diagnose*
anything would be absolutely no use to me!

The art of differential diagnosis goes to the heart of practising medicine, yet it is a skill that many clinicians rarely think
about or discuss. Think of all the worried people sitting in
the waiting area of an emergency department or GP surgery
on a Monday morning. Often, they know that they feel awful

---

enough to have felt the need to seek care, but have no way of knowing why they have that dull ache in their chest or burning pain in their stomach or persistent headache. In an ideal world, their diagnosis would be so obvious that they might as well have a Post-it note stuck to their forehead that said 'angina' or 'duodenal ulcer' or 'brain tumour' – then it would just be a matter of confirming the correct treatment and management plan.

In the real world, however, it's seldom that easy. Most diagnosis is essentially the consequence of following a virtual or actual flowchart with yes or no questions about clinical symptoms and laboratory test results until you pinpoint the disease or condition that the patient has. However, many human disease processes are simply not understood in sufficient detail to enable this level of certainty to be attained. Much clinical medicine encompasses an element of the unknown – perhaps the stage in the development of understanding of a disease when we know that 'something happens', but don't yet know what that 'something' is.

That is where good medical research comes in, finding ways to identify, question and illuminate the most urgent of the unknowns. Vast swathes of human disease fall within the realms of medically unexplained symptoms, our ignorance even labelled with the acronym 'MUS' – as if by doing so, we can take our absence of knowledge and make it into a named clinical entity (job done!). A new, uncharted disease process for which we lack bespoke, validated tests and for which the routine tests prove unilluminating, such as Long Covid, is virtually guaranteed to earn itself the MUS soubriquet.

Medically unexplained symptoms should be taken as an indication that more tests and investigations are needed, but often if standard tests don't show anything, clinicians default to thinking that the symptoms are psychological or even made up. Contemporary medical care, informed by genetic analyses and molecular technologies, looks very different from that of 100 years ago, and it is likely that in another 100 years it will have transformed radically again. Progress will be made by the willingness of curious people to fill in the knowledge gaps surrounding medically unexplained symptoms.

It is sometimes proposed that the prognosis in patients with medically unexplained symptoms is the product of three criteria: multiple symptoms, affecting multiple systems, occurring on multiple occasions. Though proposed long before the pandemic, that sounds to me like a rather good description of Long Covid.

A Dutch study showed that GPs labelled symptoms as 'medically unexplained' within two and four minutes of the start of patient consultations, depending on whether the patient had discussed the symptoms in previous consults (this reduced the time to GP conclusion).[14] The paper concluded that non-analytical reasoning was a central component in these GPs' thought processes. That is to say, the doctors were acting on instinct, and when that instinct is formed in the context of a knowledge gap and a trust gap – well, we get bias.

Now that our healthcare systems have been struggling through a pandemic for years, Sarah Graham argues that an empathy gap is also emerging among primary healthcare providers. Certainly, NHS staff have been under a huge amount of pressure, and are under-resourced and overworked. 'Compassion fatigue' is a real thing, whereby burnout leads to a reduction in the healthcare provider's ability to care for their patients in an empathetic manner.[15]

When you combine this empathy gap with the knowledge and trust gaps, you can start to see why long haulers are dissatisfied or upset with the care they've received from their healthcare providers. Given that most people with Long Covid are women, and that women with chronic illnesses are more likely to experience mini-misation, psychologisation or gaslighting, this is a hugely important issue. Before we address the challenging topic of how to challenge the status quo, let's dive into another sex-specific issue with Long Covid.

Why do women's Long Covid symptoms get worse at certain points in their cycle?

To best answer this question, I conversed with my colleague Dr Viki Male at Imperial College London. Dr Male is a lecturer in reproductive immunology, and so is extremely well placed to comment on the nature of the immune system during women's reproductive cycles. So, going back to first principles, we can roughly think of the immune system having two main types of response to invading organisms: type 1 responses mostly involve immune cells and type 2 responses mostly involve antibodies.

During pregnancy, the immune system shifts from a type 1 cellular response towards a type 2 antibody response. This means that the autoimmune diseases mediated by antibodies, such as lupus, myasthenia gravis and Graves' disease, get worse in pregnancy, whereas those mediated by cellular immune responses – such as MS and rheumatoid arthritis – tend to get better.

Now going into the menstrual cycle, we can think of the second half of the cycle after ovulation as being a lot like pregnancy. The body is preparing for pregnancy such that if there's a fertilised egg present it can implant successfully. At this time the immune system is quite similar in some ways to how it is in pregnancy, so it wouldn't be surprising if those diseases that tend to get worse in pregnancy got worse in the second half of the menstrual cycle, or if those that tend to improve in pregnancy got better.

As we've previously discussed, there is strong evidence that there is an autoimmune component to Long Covid, so we absolutely expect that the resulting symptoms would change over the course of the menstrual cycle. However, from what I've heard among the community, there doesn't yet seem to be any data or a super clear picture about when and how symptoms change, so conclusions are still hard to draw. At the time of writing, the teams at Imperial College London have just received grant funding to set up a new study to look at this in detail.

The suggestion that data about menstrual cycles might be enlightening spurred me to work. I put together a survey and shared it on social media platforms and in support groups. In total, 603 women completed the survey, of whom 570 were still menstruating. Over half of respondents (253 of 463 answering the question) reported that their cycles had changed since developing Long Covid (it had become more irregular in all but twenty-four); 421 (75%) of 563 respondents had a regular pattern of symptoms across their cycles. Of these 421 respondents, 63% reported that their symptoms changed in the approach to and during menstruation, 10% found their symptoms changing in the first half of their cycle (leading up to ovulation), and the remaining 27% reported changes in the second half of their cycle.

Almost universally, these 421 participants reported that their symptoms got worse (with 180 reporting their symptoms got slightly worse and 214 saying they got *much* worse). Only eight said their symptoms got slightly or much better. The remaining nineteen participants said their symptoms changed in nature but remained of a similar severity. The five most frequently reported worsening symptoms were:

1. fatigue/post-exertional malaise
2. headaches

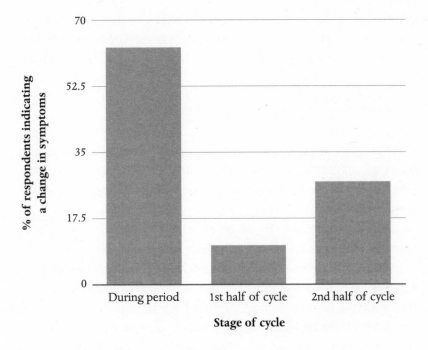

3. dysautonomic symptoms (increased heart rate, palpitations, dizziness)
4. mental health issues
5. neurological and muscular symptoms.

To summarise, my data shows that if you menstruate, it's extremely likely that your Long Covid symptoms will vary during your cycle. And, if they do, they're much more likely to get worse rather than better. In addition, your cycle itself is likely to become more irregular.

I asked Dr Viki Male for her take on these findings, and she felt that the pattern of symptoms that the survey respondents reported is consistent with other autoimmune diseases mediated by T cells (rather than autoantibodies). These autoimmune diseases tend to get better during pregnancy, but also during the twelve or so days after ovulation (when the body is preparing for pregnancy). They get worse just before the period starts and during the period. If we were to assume viral persistence in Long Covid, then this could also be in line with symptoms occurring more at times when the cellular immune response is more actively trying to control uncleared virus. Of course, these are very preliminary findings, and rigorous research is most definitely needed on this subject.

How to tackle gender bias as a patient

Prof. Hughes argues that although medical doctors don't go into medicine expressly to discriminate against women, their entire clinical world view is constructed based on a history of prejudice. Structural discrimination is, by its very nature, difficult to remove or address. Sometimes it can be difficult to even discuss because there's a strong resistance to accepting that the problem exists.

While patients shouldn't have to take steps to help themselves, until we see major systemic change it pays to take a few steps to minimise the issues they face. At the very least, if patients are aware that they might be facing unconscious bias, then they will be in a better position to avoid it or challenge it. I asked Prof. Hughes, Sarah Graham and Dr Muirhead for suggestions to help women minimise their experience of gender bias, on an individual level:

- Be as well informed as possible about the prevalence and nature of the issue – whether Long Covid or another chronic illness – as you can be.
- Be confident in your knowledge of your own body, and be confident about expressing your symptoms and knowing that they are real, significant and worthy of a doctor's attention.
- Keep a diary of your symptoms. With Long Covid, symptoms are likely to come and go – knowing when they occur and when they die down can be important.
- Make lists of objective events that show how your illness is impacting your daily life and how it is different from your life before. Go through the lists methodically and try to make your experiences as tangible and undeniable as possible for the doctor.

- Be as logical and rational as you can be when talking to the healthcare provider. If you can, remove any emotion that might give your doctor the ammunition to say, 'You're obviously anxious or depressed.'
- If you can, take someone with you for appointments who can act as an advocate, speak on your behalf or remind you if there are things you forget to mention in the heat of the moment. Even if they are present only as a witness, you can still turn to them afterwards and get a sense-check with questions like, 'Am I being unreasonable?', 'Were they a bit patronising?' or 'Were they a bit dismissive?' Anecdotally, some patients find that their doctors talk very differently to them if they're accompanied by a man.
- If you're unhappy with the care you receive, it's worth making the effort to see another doctor. It's not always easy to do, especially with limited energy, but everyone is entitled to a second opinion.
- If possible, book a double appointment. Chronic illnesses are complex and very difficult to convey in a five- or ten-minute appointment.

There is a fundamental power imbalance in the doctor–patient relationship (especially if the patient is cognitively impaired). The patient will always be on the back foot. It is possible that you might do everything right, and still your doctor won't believe you or take you seriously. If this happens, it's not your fault. Do your best to change doctor or get a second opinion. You can find more practical advice on how to help your GP help you with Long Covid in the next chapter.

What changes need to happen to start tackling the problem of gender bias on a wider societal basis? The experts had a range of thoughts:

- a move to a fifty–fifty split in time spent on teaching male- and female-orientated diseases at medical school
- more emphasis on compassion and empathy in medical teaching and in wider educational settings

- information and awareness raising in the wider community backed up by concrete data to help make this awareness stick more than intangible or vague assertions
- individuals sharing their stories and their experiences (whether on social media or other platforms) to build a powerful block of evidence
- sharing of knowledge in communities to help patients find their way to healthcare providers who understand their condition
- lobbying (if you have the energy and resources) – whether it's Parliament or the Royal College of General Practitioners.

Ultimately, anything that helps to close the knowledge and trust gaps will begin to change the status quo. The knowledge gap is perhaps easier to address (although it does require research to establish the knowledge and then time for this to permeate through the community and for medical textbooks to change), while the trust gap is more of a societal and cultural issue. Generally speaking, progress has been made in gender relations and perceptions in the past twenty years and the hope has to be that this will continue in the future.

GEZ: How frequently does gender bias affect diagnosis and treatment of chronic illness?

DR TANIA DEMPSEY: The majority of patients whom I see have a story about a difficult experience with a doctor, a nurse or another medical professional. Everyone has a story, and that's trauma, medical trauma. In turn, trauma shapes how their body heals, how their mast cells react – everything that happens to them can potentially make their conditions worse (see chapter 9). It's really disheartening when this happens, but many healthcare providers assume that the patients are making it up, exaggerating or histrionic. Men certainly get some of this (if you're chronically ill, you are inevitably going to have some bias against you). They are generally made to feel like they should just push through. In women, the problem is the assumption that they are unreliable historians in describing their pain and other symptoms. How we change it is the big question.

GEZ: How do you approach the symptom flares that come with women's monthly cycles?

DR TANIA DEMPSEY: The key is trying to figure out what will shut down the inappropriate mast cell response, which comes in reaction to changing hormone levels. Some patients don't seem to respond to antihistamines – but if you dig deeper, they might have tried six or seven of them, and it's only when you get to the eighth that you strike gold. There are no hard and fast rules for which antihistamines will work for each patient – as a result of the complexity of the disease process it's extremely difficult to predict. One essential part of this process, though, is to be systematic with the addition and deletion of medications, but this does mean it can take some time to get to the right combination.

I wish we could say to your readers, 'Oh, this is what I would try next,' but it's really so individual. Ultimately, patients need to track their cycles and symptoms and then find a specialist to discuss with.

GEZ: To what degree do medical textbooks include chronic illnesses that typically affect women?

DR NINA MUIRHEAD: Generally speaking, they don't – and there needs to be a new chapter added. Kumar and Clark are the authors of the biggest medical textbook in the UK, and I know one of them actually. I should give him a call and say, 'Right, time to update the textbook.' In fact, that would be an interesting study – to look at how much coverage is devoted to different disease subtypes in medical textbooks. For example, just a couple of pages out of thousands are dedicated to ME/CFS in all medical textbook literature.

Summary

Gender bias remains a problem in the diagnosis and treatment of chronic illness, and when you consider that Long Covid is both chronic and primarily experienced by women, the tools needed by long haulers to combat it have never been more important. Gender bias is not always obvious, but if you educate yourself about the issue and go into consultations with clinicians well equipped, then you give yourself the best chance to deal with it. Hopefully we can begin to close those knowledge and trust gaps that are responsible for the perpetuation of the problem. In the next chapter, we will address the huge subject of how Long Covid impacts mental health.

CHAPTER 7: *The Impact of Long Covid on Mental Health*

It's almost impossible to experience Long Covid without it having some kind of impact on your mental health. Anxiety and depression feature very heavily in symptom surveys of the condition, and with good reason. Long Covid has a huge impact on your quality of life. One American study found that patients with Long Covid reported low quality of life as frequently as patients with cancer.[1] That might sound dramatic to those who are unfamiliar with Long Covid, but to those who have it, it is no surprise at all.

Clinical psychologist (and long hauler) Dr Sally Riggs describes Long Covid as the one of the most difficult things that people are likely to go through in their lives. She argues that, of all the other things that you could possibly go through (including disability, loss, death of loved ones), there's pretty much nothing else out there that no one else has ever experienced. When your life is upended this dramatically, when even basic things you took for granted are suddenly removed, it is inevitable that there will be consequences for mental health, the important word here being 'consequences'. One point this chapter will strive to emphasise is the direction of causality involved. Mental health is affected in three ways:

1. directly because of serotonin and dopamine levels being affected by Long Covid[2, 3]
2. indirectly because of the huge symptom burden experienced and the resulting impact on quality of life
3. depression and other mental health problems have also been increasingly associated with chronic low-grade inflammation and microglia activation.[4]

What absolutely is *not* the case is that your Long Covid symptoms are a consequence of pre-existing anxiety or depression. You may meet doctors who tell you that they are – unfortunately attitudes like this persist. But the science clearly shows (just take a look back at chapters 4 and 5) that is extremely clear that serious biological disease processes are involved.

How common are mental health issues in other post-viral conditions?

One of the most useful resources is a recent meta-analysis (in which the results of lots of separate studies are collated so that their data can be collectively analysed) of studies on post-viral mental health problems.[5]

The authors identified fifty-nine relevant studies from around the world, including patients who had experienced Covid, SARS, MERS, Ebola virus infection and bird flu. They found that 'anxiety, depression, and post-traumatic stress, and general distress were substantial beyond the acute phase. These results show that a considerable proportion of infection survivors will suffer from mental health problems severely for a longer time.' Their analysis suggested that, overall, around a fifth of all those infected across these conditions developed considerable mental health issues in the period after epidemic viral infection. They make the point that clinical support for mental health problems following infection needs to be part of care pathways and should have been included as part of the Covid treatment package from the outset.

Before we go any further into the discussion of mental health, it's essential that we break down some of the myths that have plagued people with ME/CFS and have not yet been entirely eradicated in Long Covid. This involves a brief history of the biopsychosocial attitudes to ME/CFS that permeated the medical community over the past thirty years.

The biopsychosocial hypothesis for ME/CFS

In the late 1980s and early 1990s, a thesis grew that people who had an illness characterised by fatigue and post-exertional malaise (which we now know as ME/CFS) were experiencing false ideation about having an organic illness (that is to say, it was thought that their physical symptoms were 'in their heads').[6] The theory was that this ideation, combined with the subsequent sedentary behaviour it prompted, led to a severe case of deconditioning, which then made activity harder and created a vicious cycle leading to depression, sleep dysfunction and cognitive dysfunction. The clinicians and academics positing this theory argued that you could interrupt this vicious cycle with two interventions: graded exercise therapy (GET) and a specific type of cognitive behavioural therapy (CBT).[7]

The fundamental principle of GET is that you increase your level of exercise over time, irrespective of your symptoms. The idea was that if there was nothing biologically wrong, then GET would help 'reprogram' your brain to tolerate increasing levels of exercise. Meanwhile, the CBT was designed to challenge the false ideation of illness. The theory was that the effect of the combined treatment would be 'curative'.

In 2011, proponents of this biopsychosocial theory published the results of the now-infamous PACE (Pacing, graded Activity, and Cognitive behaviour therapy: a randomised Evaluation) trial in *The Lancet*, which suggested that GET and CBT could moderately improve outcomes in ME/CFS.[8] As a result, treatment guidelines around the world were changed to recommend GET and CBT. However, there was an outcry from patients who found that the treatments *did not* help and that GET in particular could be extremely harmful (as you will probably know if you've tried to exercise yourself out of Long Covid).[9]

The tide started to change in 2015, when the US National Institutes of Health and the National Academy of Medicine published major reports describing ME/CFS as a biological illness that was not psychological in origin.[10, 11] They were essentially debunking the PACE trial without mentioning it by name. Then David Tuller from the University of California, Berkeley published a massive takedown of the PACE trial and its flawed methodology.[12] Finally a patient called Alan Matthews managed to successfully file for the PACE data to be released. It was subsequently re-analysed, and what the patient community had suspected for years was proved: CBT and GET have no efficacy whatsoever in treating ME/CFS, and may even be harmful.[13]

The National Institute for Health and Care Excellence (NICE) guidelines for ME/CFS have been changed to no longer recommend graded exercise therapy, and CBT is no longer regarded as 'curative'. However, not all healthcare professionals are up to speed on these developments. You may encounter doctors who treat Long Covid in a similar way to how they used to treat ME/CFS. At the slightest suggestion of GET, I would advise seeking an alternative GP.

What evidence is there for dysregulation of serotonin or other neurotransmitters in post-viral conditions?

Serotonin is one of the most interesting and complex chemicals in the body, with multiple targets and roles. Much of this complexity comes from the fact that it functions both as a neurotransmitter regulating function in the central nervous system, and as a transmitter in the periphery, where it is synthesised in the gut, taken up by circulating platelets and then interacts with many immune cell types, including mast cells, monocytes and T cells. Peripheral serotonin concentrations can rise considerably in inflammation.[14]

Most people, though, are probably more familiar with the role of serotonin in the central nervous system in the regulation of depression, aggression, sleep, anxiety and psychosis. Clues to serotonin's impact on these conditions come from the fact that selective serotonin uptake inhibitors (SSRIs), which increase the amount of available serotonin, have become so prevalent as a drug treatment of depressive and anxiety disorders. But after decades of research on serotonin's role in the immune system, the picture is increasingly complex.

Lots of different immune cells have serotonin receptors, including monocytes, dendritic cells (which boost immune responses by presenting invasive antigens to other immune cells), neutrophils, mast cells, B cells and T cells. Unsurprisingly, in light of this complexity, different experimental systems show that serotonin either suppresses or enhances immune functions, such as the release of cytokines. Studies of the immune or inflammatory response in the many people prescribed SSRIs for depression or anxiety tend to emphasise that the drugs have a generally anti-inflammatory effect.

This data doesn't offer any clear or magic answers about what happens to serotonin levels in post-viral conditions, but at least it gives us some ideas about what we should be looking for.

Why is depression so rife?

Now that we've clarified exactly why Long Covid isn't merely a manifestation of anxiety or depression, let's go into some more depth on the reasons why your mental health might have taken a hammering during the past few years. We can start with the impact of the pandemic itself:

- people have lost friends, family and colleagues
- people have lost their jobs or their ability to work
- people have been isolated from their loved ones
- people have been confined to their living space during lockdowns, sometimes in difficult or abusive environments
- people who experienced serious consequences from Covid live in fear of reinfection
- the future has become increasingly uncertain and scary
- inflation is spiralling and a global recession is looming.

In addition, there is no shortage of *grief*. At some level we are all grieving the world we used to know, because it's gone and will not come back. We may hope that we regain our health, but that might be the best-case scenario – our *lives* are unlikely to be the same ever again.

Mental health issues can take a variety of forms. Rather than make an exhaustive list, I will address the primary form that most people think of (and experience) – depression.

What is depression?

The NHS lists the mental symptoms of depression, sometimes known as clinical depression, major depression or major depressive disorder, as:

- continuous low mood or sadness
- feeling hopeless and helpless
- low self-esteem
- feeling tearful
- feeling guilt-ridden
- feeling irritable and intolerant of others
- lacking motivation or interest in things
- finding it difficult to make decisions
- not getting any enjoyment out of life
- feeling anxious or worried
- having suicidal thoughts or thoughts of harming yourself.

The physical symptoms include:

- moving or speaking more slowly than usual
- changes in appetite or weight (usually decreased, but sometimes increased)
- constipation
- unexplained aches and pains
- lack of energy
- low sex drive
- changes to your menstrual cycle
- disturbed sleep.

Do any of these symptoms seem familiar? Even if they do, depression is harder to pin down than a list of symptoms. You can't look at that list and understand what someone who is experiencing depression is feeling. I say this from experience. My pre-conceived ideas of what depression was like were very different from the reality when I finally experienced it. Maybe it's like Burning Man* – you have to have gone to know what it's like. But for those of you who haven't experienced it, here's the 'party boat' metaphor I came up with to describe my personal experience of depression, and my journey into it for the first time.

For the first thirty-eight years of my life, I was – like most people I knew around me – happily riding on the top deck of a big boat. Music was playing and everyone was having a great time. I wasn't even aware it was a party boat – it was just the way things were and always had been. But then a huge amount of emotional stress came at me from every angle in my life, and was compounded by the sudden death of my mother. I held it together for a couple of months, but then fell overboard. It was my first time in the water, and I told myself that I was fine. But I wasn't, I was sinking.

At first, I could still see the boat in the distance, hear the music playing and see the people dancing on the deck. I could remember what it felt like to be up there. But as I sank underwater, the boat got blurry. The music became muffled. Remembering what it felt like to be 'normal' got more and more difficult. As I sank deeper, the boat disappeared from view, and even the rays of sunlight penetrating the depths started to fade. Eventually there was no light at all. When you get to that point, things really are bad. You can't remember what it feels like to wake up in the morning feeling normal, laugh at a joke or feel happy or content. All there is is pain.

Now here's one common misunderstanding about depression – that it's all in the head. It's not. For many (including me), it's an active, physical, churning pain that drills away somewhere deep in the gut. This pain dominates so much of your mind that your

---

* The annual festival that takes place in the Black Rock Desert in Nevada, USA.

thinking can itself becomes distorted, irrational, angry, upset or impulsive. A lot of the time, you don't even realise that you're thinking or behaving that way. It sneaks up on you. I first realised I had an issue when I was persuaded to take an online test (Beck's Depression Inventory, which I can recommend as a reasonable diagnostic tool, providing you are honest with yourself). I scored thirty-eight, indicating severe clinical depression, even as I was trying to deny I had a problem. To go back to my earlier metaphor – I was already overboard and sinking quickly.

Our experiences – or 'baggage' – drive a lot of how we react to the pain of depression. Many of us become withdrawn. Others become moody or confrontational. Self-harm might not make a lot of sense to you until you realise that, when you experience that much internal pain, the immediate relief of creating a lesser, controllable pain somewhere else becomes almost logical. One thing that you can say about depression is that there are no hard and fast rules. It's just a really, really horrible place to be.

Depression and Long Covid

I'm not a mental health professional, but what I can do is talk about how Long Covid affected me and my mental health, and about what helped me. Just before the pandemic, to extend my previous metaphor, I'd managed to get out of the water and had constructed myself a dinghy. It was moderately stable, and I was attempting to paddle my way back to the party boat, but was still some way from getting there. Fundamentally, though, I had a purpose and direction. What kept the dinghy from capsizing were two primary coping mechanisms.

The first was being *productive* (or just feeling like I was being productive): making progress, going forwards, achieving goals – even if only minor ones. The other coping mechanism was *exercise*. On average I was running an hour a day as part of my marathon training. Three of my six runs a week were extremely intense and provided massive dopamine boosts. Unfortunately, Covid and the subsequent fatigue swiped both of those coping mechanisms in one fell swoop, and the effect of losing them subsequently compounded over time.

As an aside, this is an excellent example of why CBT doesn't work in Long Covid. The behavioural activation school of CBT prescribes the 'forcing' of activity and productivity (to deliver a sense of achievement and bring about joy). But any attempt to do this during Long Covid could cause post-exertional malaise and be actively harmful.

Three or four weeks after getting Covid I realised that the sea my dinghy was floating in had got choppy: the waves were big and I was getting wet. It didn't take long until I capsized. In the absence of my coping mechanisms, a range of *feelings* contributed to this setback:

- Frustration: every day, I wanted to get on with work or other projects but felt too terrible. So, days would pass and still nothing got done.
- Failure: I felt bad about myself, not good enough.
- Crushing disappointment: some days I would wake up feeling better, and I couldn't help but get my hopes up, and try to do a little bit more. Then the next day I would be hit with brutal post-exertional symptom exacerbation.
- Selfishness: I worried that people around me might want help or assistance and that I would be unable to give it.
- Fraudulence: I didn't tell people that I was suffering, and the pressure of not talking about it grew and I felt like a fraud.
- Worry: after weeks without any progress, I worried about getting better – would there ever be another day when I would wake up without a headache?
- Uncertainty: would there be a time when I could make plans for the next day or the next week and know that I'd be able to keep them? What does recovery look like? When will it happen? How does it happen?
- Insecurity: would I be able to go for a day out and not worry about having to lie down or crash for hours in the middle of it?

- Pressure: could I handle going back to work? Could I deal with a week of 7 a.m. alarms, commuting and ten-hour work days, with life admin on top? (No way. Just one of those would wipe me out for a week.)
- Grief (and all its derivative emotions): possibly the most heavyweight of all these feelings. I would see people doing the simple things I used to love doing (exercising, social-ising) and wish that I could to do them too. But it felt a very, very long way away and I wasn't sure if I'd ever be able to do them again.

Elisabeth Kübler-Ross proposed that there are five stages of grief: denial, anger, bargaining, depression and acceptance. You may find that you go through all these feelings early in your Long Covid journey. A common myth is that you travel through the five stages linearly, but the reality is that you will find yourself bouncing between them like a pinball, or experiencing them at the same time. There was one though that, for me, lingered a long, long time. Anger.

The longer the ill health goes on, the greater the pressure builds, along with the list of undone tasks, the emptying of the bank balance with no income to replenish it. What is it like when you've got kids, or dependents of any kind? How can you care for them when you barely have the ability to get through your own day? I can't even imagine how difficult this would be.

The context to these feelings is:

1. a backdrop of global pandemic, geopolitical unrest, uncertainty and looming recession
2. an incredibly debilitating illness, with no prognosis, effective treatments or cures (yet)
3. depression as a potentially direct biological symptom of Long Covid
4. a consequential life impact with no obvious relief or light at the end of the tunnel.

The phrase has become tired, but we live in unprecedented times. Previous generations lived through world wars and were scarred by them. Mental health issues were largely brushed off at the time. We know more about them now and dealing with them before they become critical is vital.

Dealing with depression

Let's talk a bit about how to deal with depression in Long Covid. First, I'm going to describe a few things that helped me get through the darkest days, and then I'll discuss a brilliant set of psychological strategies developed by Dr Sally Riggs to help deal with the unique challenges of Long Covid. You might notice that a number of themes are shared between my thoughts and Sally's. Choose the advice that resonates best with you. So much of this experience is personal that whatever action you decide to take has to feel authentic and right to you on a fundamental level. I also recommend seeking further advice and treatment: GPs have an extensive toolkit and are used to treating depression.

PRODUCTIVITY

With depression or Long Covid – and especially when you have both – there is going to be a significant impact on what you're able to do in a day. If you're used to doing a lot, this is going to come as a shock. The first part here is acceptance: accept your new energy level. You might need to grieve the old one, but don't worry, be patient, do the right things and you can slowly build from there. Then make lists. Make them long, make them easy, and stick things on them to tick off that you've already done. I'm talking about really banal stuff here. The first thing on my daily list is 'breakfast'. That's right – every day, I get a point just for eating breakfast. Your daily list might be as simple as:

Breakfast
Take a shower
Do washing

Make lunch
Nap
Email John
Take meter readings
Reheat leftovers
Bath
Bed

Reward yourself for managing to do the things that you previously didn't even think about doing. Because with Long Covid (and with depression) these things are *hard*. Other people won't get it (unless they've had similar experiences). Be patient with them and encourage them to be patient with you. The marvel of making simple lists like this is that when you get to the end of your day and you've ticked off everything on your list, that's a 100% productive day. Reframe, and accept your limitations.

ACTIVITY/FRESH AIR

Exercise is a controversial topic in the world of Long Covid, and please be assured that I am not specifically recommending it here. Some people may find exercise helps depression, but it can be a very bad idea in any condition in which post-exertional malaise is a risk.

That said, being completely sedentary should be avoided. Try to find a comfortable low level of activity that doesn't trigger post-exertional malaise in the following days. Daylight helps regulate your circadian rhythm, and we need as much help with that as we can get, given the sleep disturbance reported by long haulers. This activity might just be having a cup of tea in the garden (if you can tolerate tea – many people with MCAS can't). Maybe you're able to walk to the shops and back. Whatever you do, stay within your limits.

One of the problems with Long Covid is that the level of activity you can manage is hard to quantify when your daily capabilities vary so much. So, if you are choosing to do something that approaches exercise, a heart rate monitor can be a useful asset. A general rule for Long Covid is that you should keep your heart rate under 60% of your maximum.[15] For those of us over the age of thirty, that means it should stay below 110 beats per minute. You might find it takes *very* little activity to get your heart rate over that mark – in which case, back off and try not to get too excited.

MEDITATION

Before Covid irrevocably changed the face of our planet, I was a bit of a meditation cynic. But since developing Long Covid, I have become a convert, and now it is one of my key coping mechanisms. If I feel the dinghy rocking a bit too much, I force myself to take five or ten minutes out and put on a meditation or breathwork app (more on this in chapter 9) – I'm not patient enough to do it by myself. After I get through the meditation (which can often be pretty hard for me, as lots of emotions come bursting out), I tend to feel much calmer and able to get on with my day – or at least calm enough to get through another couple of hours till I need to meditate again.

SLEEP

Broken or unrestful sleep is a common symptom of Long Covid. This sleep disturbance can produce various other complications, including emotional issues – if you're struggling anyway, a bad night's sleep is the last thing you need. Matthew Walker's book *Why We Sleep* is an invaluable resource that's worth well more than its cover price.[16] In it he discusses the studies that show how not getting a full night's sleep can affect our ability to regulate emotion (and everything else) and provides some simple practical actions you can take to improve sleep hygiene.

THERAPY

If you don't have the energy to make it out of the house to see a psychotherapist or counsellor, many of them will work over Zoom. Good therapy will not resolve your Long Covid, but will probably help you to cope with depression. Unfortunately, the NHS waiting lists for psychotherapy are huge, so this can be an expensive option.

SUPPORT

Talk to people you care about. You might not be able to see them in person, but give them a bell if you feel up to it – you might be surprised how much better a good phone call can make you feel. It's hard to motivate yourself to do it sometimes when all you want to do is curl into a ball, but if you know anyone who doesn't immediately clam up when you talk about feelings, give them a shout. And, finally ...

KINDNESS

Depression tends to make people withdraw and become self-focused and internalised. If you can find it in yourself to do one small random act of kindness a day, you might be surprised at the positive effect it can have – not just on the person (or animal or plant) who receives the kindness, but on yourself. It changes your state of mind, makes you look outwards and provides the kind of chemical reward that your brain is not getting enough of.

I can't really talk about mental health and depression without mentioning medication. This an absolutely huge, complex subject that ultimately is beyond the scope of this book. What I will say is that personally I benefitted from a low dose of an SSRI (escitalopram) during my Long Covid journey, and another drug (mirtazapine) has helped hugely with sleep. Speak to your doctor if you think you could benefit from medication, but bear in mind that most SSRIs take a few weeks to work. You also need to be carefully tapered off them if you decide to stop taking them.

Five psychological strategies to deal with Long Covid

Let's address Dr Riggs's five strategies to help you deal with what Long Covid throws at you.

FEEL YOUR FEELINGS

Dr Riggs argues that people with Long Covid experience many overwhelming feelings, which tend to worsen symptoms, and so, over time, many people start trying to avoid these emotional waves. Unfortunately, that isn't going to help, because suppressed emotions can lead to negative outcomes medically and psychologically.

The goal is to find a way to experience your feelings until they dissipate. One trick here is to 'observe and describe',[17] so that you can notice what's happening in your body and describe it non-judgementally – for example, 'I feel sad and it's OK to feel sad (and I'm not going to punish myself for feeling sad).' This approach extends to all feelings: it's OK to feel helpless, it's OK to feel hopeless – they will pass. By letting yourself experience those feelings, you will be able to get back sooner to where you want to be, without the additional nervous system burden of bottling it up. Dr Riggs describes how feelings like anger, sadness, bitterness and frustration usually only remain at their maximum intensity for a short period, so you can be assured that, as awful as feeling those feelings might be, they won't last for ever.

Another strategy that Dr Riggs suggests is journalling – just open up a blank Word document or notebook page when you feel overwhelming feelings and write down all your thoughts and feelings in a stream of consciousness. Write down everything, bad and good. You will notice that, as time goes on, your words will change, your feelings will change and your burden is lighter. Then delete the contents of the page so you're not tempted to revisit and ruminate.

One of the contradictions in the Long Covid experience is that it involves improvement and relapse. Once you've started to recover and some good days have given you hope, when you then have a bad day the negative feelings can be more insurmountable than they were the first time around. Then it becomes a question of trying to keep in mind those good times – almost like burning the image into your memory so that the next time you need it, you can draw on it as evidence that yes, another good day is around the corner, and you don't need to panic.

Dr Riggs describes how each time she got the Covid vaccine her symptoms seemed to worsen, and when she had the booster she was really sick for seventy-two hours. Despite the fact she'd been through the experience twice already and had had multiple non-vaccine-related relapses before this point, in that moment of feeling so terrible, it was so hard to convince her brain that what she was feeling wouldn't be for ever. She recommends channelling Guy Pearce's character with memory loss in *Memento*, who has to put Post-it notes everywhere to remind himself of what's happening, only in this scenario the notes remind you that the bad feelings will pass and it will be OK. So, taking selfies or videos when you're at your best can be a good idea – they can help to remind you when you're at your worst that it's still possible to get back to a better place.

TRUST YOUR GUT

Trusting your gut is incredibly important when navigating Long Covid. It's useful advice whether you're having your illness mini-mised by doctors and starting to question if you're really sick, making decisions about which of the 3,000 recommended supple-ments or expensive holistic treatments to invest your money in, or choosing who among your loved ones to include in your support group, or when you have conflicting pieces of advice – maybe doc-tors telling you that you need to exercise more or that you should take antidepressants. All of these experiences can be incredibly overwhelming and destabilising.

In moments like these, it's worth being still for a moment to pay attention to your body. This is where the gut instinct resides, and this is where your answer is. At a deep level, you know what you need. Perhaps if you're in the middle of a relapse and you don't feel safe, ask yourself what you need to feel safe. If you're feeling pressure to act a certain way or do certain things, ask yourself do you really want to? Is it in the best interests of your health? Sometimes (maybe much of the time) what we need to do is rest. And that's OK. Give yourself permission to listen to your gut and do what is right for you – not what other people think is right for you.

CALM THE FIGHT-OR-FLIGHT RESPONSE

We introduced the idea of the three-tier structure for the nervous system (as described by neuroscientist Dr Stephen Porges) in chapter 2, where we move from the parasympathetic response (rest, digest and heal) through to the sympathetic response (fight or flight) and in extreme cases then into immobilisation. One of the observations of long haulers is that we seem to spend a disproportionate amount of time with our sympathetic nervous systems activated (in fight-or-flight mode), which is potentially triggered by inflammation innervating the vagus nerve or by direct nerve damage. If you're in fight-or-flight mode for too long, the body may ultimately then shift into immobilisation as a self-protection mechanism. This is when your body shuts down and there's nothing you can do to get it going again. Any of us who've crashed hard and found the fatigue so overwhelming that we literally can't get out of bed have probably experienced this. How do we stop ending up here? By calming the nervous system while in fight-or-flight mode to return us to the parasympathetic response of rest, digest and heal.

Dr Sally Riggs recommends the Safe and Sound Protocol (SSP), a non-invasive passive listening therapy that plays specific types of music that help to calm the nervous system down. But there are many ways of calming the nervous system – it's a question of trying to find the methods that work for you. Breathwork and meditation can be very powerful (we'll come back to these in chapter 9). Devices that stimulate the vagus nerve can also be very effective. A range of devices at different price points are available. I have had excellent results with an 'Alpha-Stim' device – I find it helps trigger parasympathetic cues like yawning within seconds of connecting it. Pacing and rest are the simplest forms of calming your nervous system down. There doesn't have to be anything sophisticated about pacing – just making sure that you stop whatever you're doing and rest for fifteen minutes every hour can make a huge difference. It goes without saying that avoiding stress or stressful triggers, whether physical or emotional, is of critical importance to success here.

If you're trying to do yoga or deep breathing or meditation and it's not working, there may also be a layer of self-criticism that makes whatever you're trying even less likely to work (self-criticism is a sure-fire road to immobilisation). With something passive like the Safe and Sound Protocol, there is no 'doing it right'. If you are struggling with any of these techniques, something similarly passive might work best for you (note that vagal stimulators are also 'passive' in that you don't need to do anything yourself).

FIND YOUR PURPOSE

You'll struggle to achieve some of these higher-level goals if you're still stuck in fight-or-flight or immobilization mode. But once you're able to, finding something that you feel passionately about that you can do without triggering post-exertional malaise can be extremely powerful. Think about what is important to you – the old question 'What makes you get up in the morning?' Dr Riggs points out that in psychology there's a lot of talk about goals, and more recently about values-driven action (i.e. behaviour based on values you believe in, rather than on emotional instincts). Both of these approaches can fuel your recovery and help to create a framework for what you're aiming for. There are a lot of people who have become active in Long Covid advocacy on social media, for example. But whatever your purpose is, ensure it's something that you feel like you can engage with and that ideally has achievable goals. Whatever it is that you find as your purpose, it will fuel and support your recovery. Just don't overdo it!

CONNECT WITH YOUR PEOPLE

Anyone with Long Covid has probably found that their existing social, familial and professional groups have had a mixed reaction to their illness. Not everyone understands it, and not everyone is willing or able to support your needs. Even if you're one of the lucky ones who has been surrounded by supportive people, society itself and the medical community are still playing catch-up with awareness of the condition.

Either way, you may find that your social group changes as a consequence of having Long Covid. Surrounding yourself with people who don't understand the demands the condition places on you (or who are generally not sympathetic) will only drive emotional stress, and that is the last thing you need. You may find that random distant friends understand what you're going through far better – these are the people to bring closer. The fundamental lesson here is not to stick to your old social groups if they're not currently helping. While family is often family and there may not be much you can do about them (!), choose to surround yourself with people who offer the kind of support you need and not those who exhibit behaviours you don't.

Stephen Porges describes how co-regulation with other people sustains us and helps keep the body in a rest-and-digest state. This is why a continued degree of social engagement (as much as possible within your given energy limits) is highly recommended. Dr Riggs recommends thinking about all the people who you've not been in contact with recently and sending them a quick text. Then, based on the responses you get, reconfigure your close circle to include only those who completely get it. The idea is that any time you're having a social interaction you should feel safe and supported, which will continue to support your parasympathetic nervous response and your recovery.

One observation you might have made about these five lessons – the repetition of the word 'your'. So much of this is individual and personal, and the overarching theme is about tuning in to *your* individual needs.

GEZ: Could you tell me about how Long Covid affects mental health?

DR SALLY RIGGS: The strange thing about Long Covid is the path it took for most of us, such that the peak of disability didn't hit until maybe six months or a year after the acute infection. In addition, there was lots of uncertainty around whether you would recover or not, given that there was absolutely no prognosis. If you take MS as an example, it can be unpredictable but it's now a well-researched condition that affects millions of people worldwide, so at least in that scenario you can get an idea of what your disability might look like. With Long Covid, none of us knew: we were all faced with the real possibility that this could be permanent disablement, which is absolutely terrifying. The resulting grief is intense.

GEZ: Elisabeth Kübler-Ross described the famous five stages of grief. To what degree is this model accepted by psychologists and used to help patients with chronic illness?

DR SALLY RIGGS: Kübler-Ross's work was really helpful and ground-breaking at the time, but grief just doesn't progress in that nice, neat order. The way that we think about grief now is that you could be feeling anything and everything all at the same time, and that's OK – or you could be feeling nothing. We think less about the stages and focus on giving people permission to be sad and angry at the same time. You may have moments of numbness, and we try to take that into account too. That seems to fit the Long Covid experience: we can quickly change from feeling furious to sad to hopeless to helpless. Grief is a normal human experience, not a disorder that you can treat away. If you've ever had a loss, you know that it will be with you for your entire life. Long Covid isn't exactly the same, obviously, because some of us are getting function back and so then that grief isn't there any more. But I think, for all of us, our lives will be dramatically different, whatever way we come out of this. We still need to process the loss of the people we used to be and to build a new person – which, again, is talked about a lot in chronic illness, generally.

Western societies have historically been bad at processing grief, compared with other cultures that don't try to hide it away. We seem to think of grief as pathological – something to be recovered from – rather than embracing it as something normal that will be part of you for ever. In terms of the Long Covid process, a lot of us were fighting those emotions for a long time – hence the importance of just allowing those emotions to be there, whatever they are and whatever they mean.

Summary

While there is huge scope in the subject of mental health generally, the experiences that long haulers have had seem to have 'funnelled' them down a particularly similar path. Feelings of denial, anger, frustration, sadness, loss and depression are almost universal among those who have had Long Covid for months or more. If you have experienced some or all of these feelings, be assured you are not alone – these feelings are a natural and healthy reaction to the situation. I hope that the strategies outlined above are of some help to navigate your way through this particularly difficult time, because the emotional assault delivered by Long Covid can be just as intense as the physical one. For more on this subject, we will discuss the emotional journey frequently experienced by those who have Long Covid in chapter 12. Next up, though, is practical advice on how to help your GP (and everyone else) understand what you're going through.

CHAPTER 8: *How to Help Others Help You*

One of the most difficult experiences for long haulers early in the pandemic (based on my experience and the testimony of many of the other first wavers) was visiting their GPs and being met with confusion, dismissal or just an absence of meaningful care. Thankfully, the situation has changed somewhat since then, and most GP practices (in the UK at least) have at least one GP who is familiar with Long Covid. Guidelines to help GPs recognise and diagnose Long Covid have been published in the *British Journal of General Practice*.[1] But what happens if your GP isn't the practice's Long Covid specialist, you live in a country which is less familiar with Long Covid, or – heaven forbid – you're unlucky enough to have a doctor who thinks it's a psychological condition?

In this chapter we'll offer a range of advice to help you get the best care, irrespective of whether your personal doctor has experience with Long Covid. We'll also delve into the collective wisdom of the Long Covid community to get some golden nuggets of counsel regarding how to help the people in your support network get their heads around what you're going through.

Why you should see your GP

I have to admit, I was one of those who didn't bother making an appointment with their GP until over nine months into Long Covid. I figured there wasn't anything they would be able to do for me. But that was perhaps short-sighted. Professor Brendan Delaney, a GP who has had Long Covid himself, offers the following wise advice for why you should see your GP:

- The symptoms of Long Covid overlap with those of several other potentially serious conditions, such as cancer, cardiac disease, kidney disease, hypothyroidism and anaemia, which all need to be ruled out.

- In the first three to six months of Long Covid, there are some rare nasty acute complications, such as stroke, cardiovascular disease and pulmonary embolisms. These complications can have specific signs or symptoms that might be caught early by a GP.
- Baseline investigations could establish whether you have dysautonomic issues such as PoTS (e.g. an active stand test, in which a jump in heart rate of thirty beats per minute between lying down and standing indicates PoTS) or have mast cell issues (e.g. by testing for Darier's sign, whereby the clinician rubs a skin lesion on the patient's arm to see if the skin reacts strongly, which can suggest overactive mast cells).
- Treatment can be prescribed, which could make a massive difference to your quality of life. For example, ivabradine or beta blockers could be given for PoTS, and antihistamines for symptoms related to MCAS.
- GPs can issue fit notes to help inform your employer of your ability to work, and they can also sign sick notes.
- GPs can also help with any mental health issues resulting from Long Covid (there is a well understood and established care pathway for mental health in primary care).
- There are efforts in the UK and elsewhere to establish specialist Long Covid clinic care pathways, but you will need a referral to access them.

How to help your GP help you

This guidance comes courtesy of three doctors who work in primary care and have personally experienced Long Covid: Prof. Delaney, Dr Susannah Thompson and an American healthcare professional. They are thus uniquely placed to advise on the best way to get the most out of your trip to the doctor. (If you are a GP looking for advice on how to manage patients, then Prof. Delaney and Dr Thompson have provided a brilliant peer-to-peer list of best practice in the Resources section on page 285.)

BEFORE THE APPOINTMENT

- Make a list of your symptoms and how often you experience them. Prioritise those that have the most impact on your day-to-day life by putting them at the top of the list.
- Quantify your symptoms if possible. For example, the symptom 'I'm exhausted' could be quantified by describing how many hours of sleep you require each night now compared with how many you needed pre-Covid. Other examples might include how many days of work you have missed in the past month, how many steps you are able to take each day before needing to lie down, and which activities you are no longer able to engage in.
- Write down the questions you have and take the list in with you.
- Ask if there's a particular GP at the practice with experience of treating Long Covid.
- Consider sending an email in advance with a list of your symptoms and what you'd like to talk about. If your GP practice uses e-consult then it will automatically go into their records. If they're not familiar with Long Covid, you might also want to point them to an excellent resource in the *British Journal of General Practice* (see the Resources section on page 283).

DURING THE APPOINTMENT

- Show your symptom list and priorities to the GP. Agree with the GP at the beginning which problem or problems can be dealt with in the appointment. They might have different priorities from you: fatigue might be your main symptom but the GP might suggest that chest pain is the most important one to check first as a serious cause might need to be ruled out.

- If there's a suspicion you might have PoTS, the PoTS UK website is an excellent resource to steer your GP to (and get information for yourself).
- GPs are experienced at dealing with many of the symptoms caused by Long Covid, including pain, vertigo, tinnitus (ringing in the ears) and fatigue. If you have any of these, it is definitely worth mentioning them.
- If you struggle with cognitive dysfunction, take someone with you who can remind you of anything you forget to mention and can remember on your behalf what the GP said. If you go alone, ask the GP to write any advice down so you don't have to remember it.

GENERAL TIPS

- Some GP practices in England have 'care navigators', who can direct patients to useful resources and various services to support other aspects of life and complement the care provided by the primary care team. This can include diet and lifestyle support, signposting to voluntary and other support groups and linking with social prescribing, whereby activities and support in the community can be used to support recovery. Don't be afraid to ask to speak to them if the practice offers the service.
- Ask to be referred to a Long Covid clinic, but expect the GP to do a number of baseline tests on you first to rule out any of the potential severe complications mentioned previously.
- GPs are used to managing unexplained symptoms and working out possible treatment options and causes, so it pays to work with them through their process. Let the doctor feel their way through the problem with you via their own questioning rather than hitting them immediately with, 'I've got all these symptoms and I'm sure I've got blood clots,' for example.

- Request to see another GP if you're not happy.
- Ask how long your visit will be so that you have an idea of how much you'll reasonably be able to discuss. If you only have a standard ten-minute slot, to get most out of the time:
  - tell your doctor up front that you're having multiple symptoms
  - give a brief overview (one or two minutes) of the course of your illness
  - agree on which of the most bothersome symptoms to discuss in detail, as time allows
  - ask if you can schedule several appointments in a short timeframe – perhaps two more across three weeks, as it is not possible to go through a complex condition like Long Covid in just one appointment.

Here's an example of how to start off: 'I tested positive for Covid on January 12, 2021. I was only mildly ill, and was not hospitalised, but ever since I've been experiencing fatigue, headaches, insomnia and rashes [show your list]. The headaches are bothering me the most right now, so I'd like to talk about those first, and I'd like to schedule a follow-up visit to discuss my other concerns.'

Healthcare providers (at least in the mainstream sector) are generally trained to evaluate their patient's symptoms by gathering a standard set of information in an organised fashion, so that they can easily compare the characteristics of the complaint to known diagnoses and rule out other diagnoses. Patients can greatly reduce the amount of time it takes to convey this information to their doctor by translating their experience into the same format in which the doctor has been trained to think. There are a few acronyms which are used to investigate symptoms (or pain), such as SOCRATES:

S: Site of the symptom (where is it?)
O: Onset (when did it start? did it come on acutely or gradually?)

C: Character (what does the symptom feel like – dull, stabbing, aching, etc.)

R: Radiation (does the sensation travel to another region?)

A: Associations (are there any other signs or symptoms connected to it?)

T: Time course (does the symptom happen at certain times?)

E: Exacerbating factors (does anything make the symptom better or worse?)

S: Severity (how bad is the symptom on a scale of one to ten?)

If you've already decided that you'd like to focus this appointment on your headaches, then ahead of the appointment break them down in this way and bring your answers with you. This will help cut down on the amount of time spent eliciting the information and leave more time for discussion of evaluation and treatment options. It would also be worth doing the same for your other most concerning symptoms in case you have time to address them in the appointment too – worst-case scenario, if you don't get to it, you can leave the symptom list and details with your GP and it may prompt them to consider your condition after you've left.

It is also worth keeping a diary of your most concerning symptoms (see page 284 in the Resources section for an example).

Why is the future of healthcare for Long Covid brighter than it has been with other post-viral illnesses?

I do see the future as brighter, and I very much anticipate that this will in turn catalyse progress in healthcare for other patient groups, especially people with ME/CFS. The praise for this brighter future should go almost entirely to the incredible efforts of the Long Covid community and support groups around the world. I'm aware that, to them, the progress of the past two years has felt painfully slow. But to me, used as I am to the glacial pace of initiatives in clinical medicine and medical research, it feels like things have been moving at lightning speed.

I wouldn't have imagined that a new disease entity would be described not in lecture theatres at the Royal Societies, but in Facebook groups and social media posts, and that within a matter of months there would be funding for NHS Long Covid clinics and then major funds for research programmes both in the UK and in the USA. The big challenge now, as policymakers try to move along from all things Covid, is to keep Long Covid on the healthcare agenda. If, as we believe, the UK alone has some 2 million people (and rising) with Long Covid, that's an awful lot of healthcare to deliver.[2]

How to help the people around you understand what you're going through

If you have Long Covid, you've almost certainly found yourself trying to describe what it feels like more times that you can count, and the odds are that, however you've tried to describe it, you haven't been able to do it justice. Because the reality is that Long Covid is like little else we've experienced in our lives. If you've not had it (or a similar chronic illness like ME/CFS), then there's very little frame of reference.

Ultimately a lot of the time it comes down to the empathy levels of the people around you. The people who you thought beforehand would understand, usually do. Those who don't stick their neck out for other people are unlikely to be any different now. But there are a few tools that you can use to help people understand that Long Covid isn't just feeling a bit tired or rundown. Diagrams are useful for visualising the complexity and severity of Long Covid, and for emphasising that the pathology is real. They can help people get to grips with the condition.

The multi-system impact of Long Covid[3]

Systemic
- Fatigue
- Post-exertional malaise

Pulmonary
- Dyspnea (breathlessness)
- Ground glass opacities
  (signs of fibrosis and
  inflammation)
- Hypoxemia
  (low blood oxygen)
- Reduced diffusion
  capacity (inefficient
  transfer of gas from
  lungs to blood)

Endocrine
- Diabetic ketoacidosis
  (high levels of ketones
  make blood too acidic)
- Mild thyroiditis
  (inflammation of
  thyroid gland)

Gastrointestinal
- Diarrhoea
- Loss of appetite

Haematologic
- Thrombosis
  (blood clots)

Neuropsychiatric
- Anxiety
- Depression
- Insomnia
- Brain fog (impaired
  attention, concentration,
  memory)

Ears-Nose-Throat
- Sore throat
- Dry cough

Cardiovascular
- Non-specific chest pain
- Myocarditis
  (inflammation of
  heart muscle)
- Palpitations
- High heart rate

Renal
- Acute kidney injury
  (sudden inability to filter)

Dermatologic
- Alopecia (hair loss)
- Rashes

Musculoskeletal
- Muscle ache
- Joint pain

I asked the online Long Covid community for suggestions on the most effective ways of helping the people around them understand the complexity and intensity of the condition. First, an analogy can be very powerful:

> *You are like an old battery that no longer fully charges when plugged in, with some special days where it magically has charged, and other days when it has to stay plugged in to do anything at all, or suddenly goes flat out of nowhere.*
> – Laurie Schram

> *It's like you've just finished a hard set at the gym and your limbs have gone into spaghetti mode – but all we did was chop some veg or change the bedsheets.*
> – Laurel J

> *I'm like an 80-year-old grieving for their 20s (even though I'm neither of those ages)*
> – Lambert Crest

Quantifying the experience can also be illustrative:

> *People seem to get it when I talk about 'usable hours', e.g. I have 3 usable hours a day and that needs to cover everything you would do in 14.*
> – Lucy Walker

> *Be specific – the number of hours I sleep every day (16–20). How long I can stand and do tasks for (5 minutes). This has helped with the 'everyone gets tired' BS.*
> – BlueDiamond

> *You never know how much energy tokens any activity might cost. Some days a shower might be 3 tokens, another day 9. There's no reason why some days you only get 5 tokens to spend when another day might be 10. Overspending is a disaster.*
> – Mandy

There are also hidden challenges that other people might not have considered:

> *The fact that cognition is draining – anything that requires focus takes energy and given you don't have much to begin with, conversation or watching TV can be draining very quickly.*
> – Olivia

> *Don't applaud me for doing things when I feel relatively well. Not doing things because I also need to pace when I feel well is infinitely more difficult, but also infinitely more beneficial for my health.*
> – HannekeZ

> *Explain that smiling, being optimistic and not complaining about symptoms does not mean that you're OK.*
> – Troy Roach

However, even with the best will in the world it's an uphill battle:

> *Accept that some people won't ever understand, and it's a drain on physical and emotional energy trying to convince them.*
> – Carol Bruce

That doesn't mean that we shouldn't try to help people understand what we're going through – it's simply that we have to be aware that our emotional energy is just as precious as our physical energy, and we need to be careful when and how we spend it. Ultimately, though, the better the people in our support networks understand what we can – and can't – do, and where we need help, the less alone we'll be on this particularly stormy journey.

GEZ: In a perfect world, what are the investigations that you would do in a patient presenting with Long Covid symptoms?

PROF. DELANEY: Dysautonomia can be adequately diagnosed using an active stand test – it doesn't require a full tilt-table test. Tilt tables may be needed to tease out a type of dysautonomia that's not PoTS for patients who are not responding to treatment. Beyond looking for Darier's sign (which not all GPs are familiar with) there are not diagnostic tests for mast cells – it's a clinical diagnosis made through interpretation of symptoms. For pain and breathlessness, a full pulmonary function test with transfer factor (to measure how your lungs take up oxygen from the air you breathe) is probably the most important investigation, but it's one that GPs can't do. GPs can measure basic pulmonary function but we can't measure the transfer factor, which teases out the small pulmonary embolisms that might otherwise get missed. On the cardiac side, I think the jury is out as to whether having mild myocarditis (inflammation of the heart muscle) or mild scarring diagnosed is going to make a difference in treatment. However, until we know that is completely benign, I would want to investigate patients and identify them. Cardiac MRIs are probably the biggest issue. There's a massive argument going on because it's an expensive and difficult investigation to do, and whether the results will actually change disease management is unclear. But I think that people do need to know if their heart has been affected by Covid.

I would add that there's more that we're hoping to be doing more widely by the middle of 2023, including fluorescence microscopy (which is used to observe fine detail of molecules within cells – or in this case to identify clots in the blood). I think microclots are one of those things that, if you look for them, you'll find in lots of people. The questions are whether there's a difference in the number of microclots between people with Long Covid symptoms and those who had acute Covid but no long-term symptoms, and whether they're on the causal pathway for Long Covid or a side effect related to immune dysfunction and endotheliitis. To me that's a massive research issue that's probably not immediately useful for clinical practice. The test that I would like to see done more widely is some form of routine platelet testing, because overactive platelets are probably a bigger problem than the microclots.

GEZ: How do you get referred to a Long Covid clinic?

DR THOMPSON: Long Covid clinics will vary by location. In England, there should be access to a Long Covid clinic for everyone, from children through to adults.

For those who have been in hospital, especially those who have been in an ICU, they will usually be referred to a post-Covid clinic via the hospital team. For those who do not fall under the care of a hospital team or were never hospitalised, GPs will do some initial testing and assessment and then refer into the Long Covid clinic as appropriate. Long Covid or post-Covid clinics should be staffed by a multidisciplinary team, including a health professional who should have access to relevant diagnostics, an occupational therapist, a physiotherapist and a psychologist, and should have access to specialists who can provide specialist diagnostic services.

The funding is limited, and realistically the clinics vary in staffing and services offered. Some Long Covid clinics are GP-led and they're very good. Some clinics are more led by occupational therapy and psychotherapy, which means that you might still need to ask your GP to consider what the physical problems are and to refer you to the appropriate specialist if it isn't available via the Long Covid clinic. For some symptoms, there might already be effective referral pathways. For example, if you have new allergy symptoms or joint problems, it might be more appropriate for your GP to refer you to an allergist or rheumatologist than to the Long Covid clinic.

GPs are picking up on other conditions like thyroid problems, diabetes and cancers, and it's really important that they do those screening tests first, to rule out anything else. There are so many things that can mimic Long Covid symptoms, and it's important to not miss anything.

GEZ: How geographically consistent is access to Long Covid clinics?

DANNY: That would be a really good topic for a social media-based survey, and of course not just in the UK. I get very incomplete feedback from colleagues on the one hand, and then see patients on social media on the other. Based on this, the picture I then put together is that there are some outstanding centres of excellence led by consultants who sprang into action to craft a service that can offer some real help, based on specialist, system-based approaches to symptoms. Meanwhile, I'm also to some extent aware of parts of the country where people are very dissatisfied and feel they were offered little more than therapeutic approaches to 'learn to live with it'. I know there are also regions where long waiting lists or lack of provision mean that it's hard to get to see anyone at all (though of course a really good GP can often help a fair amount). We so urgently need to look at best practice and work out the costings, personnel, specialties and equipment that we need to have in place, how much of it we need and whereabouts we need it.

Summary

Although no two people with Long Covid have quite the same experience, one of the more universal constants is the struggle to communicate to others how challenging and debilitating the condition really is. This is not necessarily a failure of communication, though – part of the problem is the ever-changing, nebulous nature of the illness itself and the difficulty of understanding the severity of some of the hallmark symptoms (e.g. fatigue, post-exertional malaise, cognitive dysfunction) if you've not experienced them.

If you're a long hauler, then analogy, quantification and visual resources can be extremely helpful to assist the people in your support network to get a handle on the slippery nature of the condition. And, when visiting your doctor, a little pre-planning can go a long way to ensure you get the best care possible. In the next chapter we'll address the top eight tips for managing the condition. You might be surprised at the difference they can make.

CHAPTER 9: Tips for Managing Symptoms

In this chapter I will discuss best practices for managing Long Covid symptoms. Note that these eight tips are lifestyle-related things you can do (or avoid) as opposed to specific treatments or medication, which will be discussed in the next chapter. As a result, you might look at the list and think it appears a bit 'soft', but in my personal experience and in that of many long haulers I've spoken to, you shouldn't underestimate the difference that adopting these can have on your wellbeing. These tips are borne out of practical experience of managing the condition for over two years and the interviews and research I have done during that time. They should not be interpreted as medical advice from a medical professional (because I am not a medical professional!). Danny will give insight and context where he judges it appropriate, though.

1. Rest

Rest is often overlooked in modern societies, but is crucial in Long Covid. There are two aspects to the role of rest – night and day. Let's start with night.

Hypersomnia (the need to sleep significantly more than usual, particularly during the day) has long been associated with post-viral conditions.[1, 2] More recently, it has also been associated with Long Covid.[3] I'd put a firm wager on the fact that if you have Long Covid you now need more sleep than you used to if you want to have even the slightest chance of functioning. 'Unrestful' sleep is one of the most cited symptoms of the condition, whereby people wake up in the morning feeling absolutely exhausted. This isn't helped by the fact that sleep can be hard to come by – many long haulers also report insomnia and disrupted sleep patterns.

There seem to be two possible reasons for this. First, dysfunction of the hypothalamic–pituitary–adrenal axis (HPA axis) has been reported in ME/CFS,[4] and I contend that the same thing could be happening in some people with Long Covid, given the similarities between the two conditions. What does this mean? In simple terms, the body's control of glucocorticoids (stress hormones that curb inflammation and manage how your cells use energy) is disrupted, leading to either lower absolute levels or release at inappropriate times. When you wake up in the morning, you would normally experience a spike in cortisol levels (to get you going), but sometimes in people with ME/CFS, this spike happens later in the day, or at much lower levels.

The second cause of unrefreshing sleep in long haulers is probably due to the nature of the sleep itself. Based on my discussions with the Long Covid community, it seems that long haulers appear to get less deep sleep than they did beforehand. Generally speaking, sleep can be broken up into two types – rapid eye movement (REM) sleep, during which you dream, and non-REM sleep, during which you enter deep sleep. According to Matthew Walker, author of *Why We Sleep*,[5] a lack of non-REM sleep leads to several negative outcomes:

- metabolic waste doesn't get flushed from the brain
- production of growth hormone is reduced, which can lead to endothelial weakness (compromising the lining of the blood vessels)
- triggering of the parasympathetic nervous system, which helps to calm the body into a 'rest, digest and heal' state, is reduced
- the ability to process new information and form memories is decreased.

This sounds rather familiar, doesn't it? I've lost count of the number of long haulers I've spoken to in whom the primary manifestations of cognitive dysfunction are the ability to process and store information, or to remember things that have happened during the course of their illness.

So why might people with Long Covid not be getting enough non-REM sleep? As discussed in chapter 7, we know that serotonin levels are affected by Long Covid. Serotonin is a precursor to melatonin, the hormone responsible for control of the sleep–wake cycle, and it stands to reason that melatonin production would consequentially be affected. The down-regulation and dysregulation of the HPA may result in inappropriate adrenal function, which interferes with natural circadian rhythms, and a body that's still in fight-or-flight mode (i.e. sympathetic nervous system activation) will also struggle to calm down sufficiently to reach deep sleep.

You may notice in Long Covid not only that you need more sleep than you used to, but also that your resilience when you get less than this ideal amount is severely compromised. Even just getting an hour's less sleep than usual can leave you in a right state the next day. So, what should you do about it?

First, prioritise sleep. Schedule time for it and don't expect to keep to the same routine you had before you were ill. The early part of the night is when we naturally get the most non-REM sleep. If we go to bed late and then sleep in, you might think it's just the same as a normal night's sleep. However, the way the body works you'll have sacrificed non-REM sleep for REM sleep. Given that we seem to be critically low on the former, this isn't a good idea. The next tip here for devising a new sleep routine is that it pays to go to bed earlier to give yourself the best possible chance of maximising your non-REM sleep.

Sleep hygiene (what you do in the hours leading up to bedtime and managing your sleep environment) is also very important. In my experience, calming the nervous system before going to sleep can pay dividends: breathwork, meditation (discussed shortly) or use of a vagal nerve stimulator (discussed in the next chapter) can help you get to sleep and reach the non-REM stage sooner. I also take a melatonin supplement around an hour before bedtime.

Let's move on to the day part of the rest equation. Perhaps you never used to factor rest into the time you spent awake – most of us do that when we're sleeping, after all. The unfortunate truth is that people with Long Covid need to factor time for rest into their days. The fatigue that long haulers face exists on a spectrum, and at the severe end people may need to spend literally all day in bed. But for those who are further along the spectrum and capable of *some* activity, there will still need to be some deliberate periods of rest. What's also worth clarifying is that low-intensity activities like having a chat, reading or watching TV do not constitute rest. These activities may not have felt like they used up energy before, but now they use up a precious amount that you may not be able to spare. Rest means just that – you are actually resting. How much rest you will need in your day (and how often) will depend on where you are on that fatigue spectrum on any given day, and the size of your energy envelope (more on this in the next section). It can be helpful to keep a very simple log detailing the number of hours' sleep you get across each day and a rating out of ten for how you feel. You are likely to see a distinct correlation between these two datasets. If you also note the three symptoms that bother you the most each day, you may be able to identify the ones that are most associated with lack of rest. It won't always just be fatigue.

2. Do less, or else ...

It might be counter-intuitive to all the health advice you've heard before, but doing *less* really is of critical importance in Long Covid. How do you work out where to cap your level of activity? Through a concept known as the 'energy envelope' (originally developed by the ME/CFS community). This isn't the kind of envelope you put a stamp on – it's the kind of envelope that it's a very bad idea to *push*. Your energy envelope is essentially the total amount of energy you can spend on any given day. You'll know if you exceed that amount because anywhere from twenty minutes to forty-eight hours later (but most commonly the next morning) you'll experience post-exertional malaise (commonly known as PEM). Post-exertional malaise feels a bit different for everyone, and can be characterised by any of the 203 symptoms mentioned back in chapter 1, but it's safe to say that if you're experiencing it, you'll know. One common – but not universal – feature is absolutely crushing fatigue, like nothing you've ever experienced before. I've previously described it as like being run over by a truck – and then chloroformed. For some there may also be headaches, joint pain, skin rashes and shortness of breath. One common factor seems to be systemic inflammation. The general rule is – do too much and the next day you have to deal with a world of pain.

Christine Miserandino introduced the 'spoon theory' to describe the experience of chronic illness.[6] The basic principle of spoon theory is that you have a limited number of spoons (say twelve) to spend on activities during the day, and each activity costs a certain number of spoons – having a shower might cost one spoon, an hour-long Zoom call might cost three, grocery shopping might cost another three. It's important to recognise that the spoon cost of activities differs from person to person. Zoom calls are my own personal journey to Hades, whereas I can tolerate driving for the same period of time no problem. Other people who have problems with visual processing may have the opposite experience. Critical to the idea of spoon theory is that you don't spend more spoons than you possess to get you through the day.

Another way of looking at the energy conundrum is that you have a battery, much like your phone or any other appliance. When you're healthy, you would normally wake up with 90–100% of your battery and could happily get through a normal working day having only spent 60% of the capacity. Perhaps the activities of daily living (showering, shopping, dealing with kids, going to the post office, etc.) use up 30% and work another 30%. The remainder you could fritter away by going to the gym or out for drinks. You probably still wouldn't have completely emptied the battery by the time you got to bed. Now imagine that you start your day with a battery that's only 25% charged. You can't even get through your normal daily activities without overspending, never mind working. As a result, somewhere, somehow, you have to make some compromises.

Some long haulers who haven't worked out where their energy envelopes begin and end exist in a constant state of post-exertional malaise, which constitutes the majority of their Long Covid experience. If they could just do less, they might find that many of their symptoms would abate. However, in the early weeks and months of Long Covid, this is difficult to accept. We are used to having a certain level of activity that we've been capable of our whole lives, usually with only occasional bouts of convalescence due to the odd virus or similar. But the cruelty of Long Covid is that this convalescence period is substantially extended and our limits drastically reduced until we recover. For most post-long haulers, this means that exercise is completely out of the question, and huge compromises have to be made elsewhere too. The emotional impact of this is massive, and is one of the primary drivers of grief (see chapter 7).

Key to managing your energy budget (whether you think of it as an envelope, a handful of spoons or a battery) is identifying the symptoms that correspond with post-exertional malaise for you. You won't know if you've overdone it until you can differentiate 'normal' Long Covid from Long Covid that has been exacerbated by post-exertional malaise. Next you need to work out which activities are particularly draining for you, which is highly individual. One thing to be aware of here is the burden of cognitive effort. It might not be something you've particularly considered in your previous life, but now you absolutely have to. This includes everything from dealing with emails and consuming online content to phone calls, Zoom calls and active processing or creative tasks. Given how variable our days can be, it can be difficult to identify which activities and which symptoms are linked. One suggestion is to extend the log mentioned in the last section: note down the primary activities in your day and how long you spent doing them, and then see if you can spot a correlation with consequential symptom burden in the next day or two.

One of the great challenges in managing our energy budgets is that the rules of the game are constantly shifting, and our post-exertional malaise limit can shift wildly from one day to the next.

Equally an activity you tolerate on one day might destroy you the next. Professor Paul Garner is now a controversial figure in the community (due to claiming that he recovered as a consequence of 'positive thinking' and exercise), but he hit the nail on the head in one of his early Long Covid articles when he likened the experience to being followed by phantom speed cameras.[7] You don't know what the speed limits are or when the harsh penalties will arrive, but arrive they will. Ultimately the best you can do is feel out your limits (exceedingly) gently and try not to spend your whole energy budget each day, because the risk that the limit will have mysteriously been lowered behind your back is quite high and not worth taking.

3. Pacing

Pacing is one of the key skills you need to develop to avoid getting sent straight to PEM jail, without passing Go or collecting £200. Have you experienced a boom-and-bust cycle with your Long Covid experience so far? If you have, you'll find that pacing is an essential tool to minimise the chances of crashing on a frequent basis.

There are a few different components to pacing, and the first we've already covered: *do less*. The next few involve *how* you do what you do. We'll break up this next part – *do differently* – into three constituent elements, the first of which is to do what you do *slower*.

We might be used to dashing about in our daily lives, multi-tasking whenever possible to keep up with the modern pace of living, never a spare moment 'wasted'. This is a concept that needs to go in the bin when you have Long Covid. It helps to do one thing at a time, and to measure the pace you do it at. A heart rate monitor can be helpful for this. It's not uncommon for your heart rate to be at a moderate level at the start of an activity and then climb quickly despite the activity not increasing in intensity – before you know it, you might be overdoing it. For example, last weekend I washed my car, which took about twenty minutes in total. For the first ten, my heart rate was below 100 beats per minute, but then it quickly climbed past 120 and 130, and by the time I'd finished it had peaked at 150. This is classic dysautonomia, and I paid the price when my post-exertional malaise showed up about twelve hours later.

What I should have done was slowed the pace at which I was carrying buckets of water and the whole car washing procedure to keep my heart rate below a sensible limit. Professor Todd Davenport, an ME/CFS specialist at the University of the Pacific in California, recommends a conservative heart rate limit of 0.55 times your maximum (which is normally calculated as 220 minus your age) for people with Long Covid or ME/CFS. I am forty-three, so my heart rate cap is around ninety-seven beats per minute. It's quite possible that this cap would have ruled out the washing the car altogether, but I could have tried to wash it slower and I would have got farther through the activity before my heart rate started rocketing.

What I should also have done is *break the activity up*. This is probably the most important single takeaway from the lesson on pacing. Had I washed half the car, come inside to lie down for ten minutes, then got up and completed the job, it is highly likely I would have managed to do the whole thing without being stung by post-exertional malaise twelve hours later.

Breaking the activity up also applies to combinations of actions that we might normally take in our day. It might be normal to get up, shower, dress and make breakfast all as a single piece in your mental to-do list. However, depending where on the spectrum of fatigue and dysautonomia you are, you may need to take a rest between each of these activities. How long that rest is will depend on the individual, but don't think that sitting down and doomscrolling on your phone constitutes rest, because it doesn't. In each of these rest periods our goal is to remove as many stimuli as possible, and to try and let the sympathetic nervous system calm down.

Travel can be very difficult to manage when you have severe fatigue, and it can be challenging to break up journeys, especially when using public transport. In these scenarios, it is helpful to leave time for a significant rest break at both ends – before you leave the house, and before you have to arrive wherever you're going – as the

Tips for Managing Symptoms

combination of rushing about, getting your stuff together, travelling and then going straight into a social engagement (or something else energy-consuming) at the other end is a recipe for disaster. By sandwiching the travel with rest you'll have a better chance of getting through the day without incident.

One thing you'll be realising at this point is that the old schedules you used to keep will no longer apply. Unfortunately, with Long Covid, everything takes longer. This is just another one of those things we have to accept.

The final element of *do differently* is to *modify your practices*. In the simplest of terms, this involves minimising the amount of time you spend standing up. Do you really need to be standing to have a shower, or to boil an egg? The answer is 'no': shower stools take some of the burden off your body while you're raising your body temperature with hot water and creating more autonomic challenges in the bathroom, and having a stool that you drag round the house and perch on when egg-boiling or doing other tasks can make a big difference too. Also consider the means of transport you choose. Perhaps you are orthostatically challenged (i.e. not tolerant of standing up for long periods) but do not find visual processing too difficult. In such a scenario driving for twice as long might be preferable to a faster but schlep-tastic experience on public transport. The key here is looking at the activities that challenge your body and trying to mitigate them, even if it's not possible to break them up or do them slower.

There are of course several barriers to effective pacing. Life is full of obligations – cooking, cleaning, working, managing relationships. It's almost certain that you will need to find compromise on at least some of these fronts. But more often than not the activities of daily living still need to be done whatever the circumstances. If you are a parent, it's very difficult getting younger children to understand what your needs might be, and the responsibility for care puts a lot on your shoulders.

Prof. Davenport points out that many people with Long Covid do not have a supportive social environment to enable pacing. In the

167

eyes of many peers, you don't just have a symptom, you have a social ill, derived from the association of fatigue with laziness or craziness, and no one wants to support those.

Some of the barriers to pacing are internal. Guilt is a hugely powerful emotion. Ruth Ainley, a clinical specialist respiratory physiotherapist in the NHS, says that she sometimes suggests to her patients that they stop doing everything (or only do absolutely essential activities) to establish a new baseline. Once the patients have been given permission to stop, a huge barrier is removed and a weight lifted. The stigma of inactivity is that powerful.

One barrier that might be a surprise is the 'good day'. When you have a good day, the temptation to catch up with everything that has been backing up can feel irresistible, but on days like these pacing is, if anything, even more essential. The number of crashes experienced by long haulers after doing too much on a good day must be getting pretty close to the number of stars in the sky. One general rule for good days is to do 50% of what you feel like you're able to and see how you get on. If you suffer post-exertional malaise afterwards, it won't be anything like as bad as it would have been without the 50% limit, and you can revise the good day target downwards for the future. If you get away with it, consider pushing the limit up gently.

Pacing is a real skill. It takes discipline, understanding from those around you and a degree of patience that might be difficult given the mental and emotional burden of your particular symptom constellation. But ultimately, unless your Long Covid is very mild indeed, pacing is a necessity rather than a choice. As time goes on, you will likely find that your energy budget increases and your subsequent need to pace decreases – but this improvement is unlikely to happen without pacing.

4. Diet

We all know that a good diet leads to better health outcomes, but before we experienced Long Covid we might not have appreciated the degree to which diet can have a massive impact on our well-being. This is the point at which my opinion and Danny's takes on the subject diverge. For context, nowhere is the chasm between evidence-less claims and mainstream medicine more apparent than in the world of fad diets and nutritional advice. If you imagine a spectrum with these fad diets at one end, and widely accepted science at the other, then the world of anti-inflammatory and low- or no-histamine diets (about which I will quote the findings from my patient-led research in this section) exist somewhere between the two. At the moment, while there is published science linking MCAS and histamine intolerance,[8, 9] it has not yet reached the degree of widespread acceptance in the scientific community. It is from this perspective that Danny offers his thoughts.

Why might managing diet help symptoms?
I have to say that some of the discussions that have gained traction among Long Covid groups, like low-histamine diets, have no resonance for me as an immunologist. That is, I can't conceive of a dietary approach that could modulate mast cell activation. My only contribution to the dietary debate is based on my previous discussion of the role of the microbiota, the incredibly diverse microcosm of bacterial species living in your gut, in inflammatory pathways. A high-fiber, low-fat diet promotes a microbiota population that tends to be anti-inflammatory and beneficial in a range of autoimmune and inflammatory conditions (a high-fat, low fibre diet could have the opposite effect).

At a mechanistic level, this is far more robust and researched than generic diet advice like 'muesli is better for your health than a full English'. The way to think about it is that your microbiota eat what you eat. If you feed them good materials, they'll metabolise these into short-chain fatty acids that exert a calming, regulatory influence over inflammatory responses around your body. If you don't, you may develop a skewed, simplified, dysregulated microbiota, which will metabolise the raw material you feed them into pro-inflammatory signals that could exacerbate inflammatory diseases at distant sites around the body, such as in the joints or the brain.

I'm certainly interested in the wave of anecdotal evidence that there is a subset of patients who report benefit from self-medicating with over-the-counter antihistamines. While I was aware that antihistamines are part of the STIMULATE-ICP trial (discussed in more detail in chapter 13), which should really help with some answers, I found myself more or less agnostic, till there's more evidence, on mast cell activation. In particular, I must confess I was especially sceptical about the ability of 'antihistamine' diets to modulate immunity. Though I've published to some extent on mechanisms in allergic disease, I suddenly wondered if there was a whole emergent branch of the subject for which I'd somehow missed the key publications? I contacted seven of the top allergists in the world and asked them about the role of histamine and the ability to modulate it through diet. They all replied fairly speedily that they were aware of no compelling evidence in support of this – that is, no pathway through which dietary modulation could be envisaged.

With Danny's thoughts on the subject duly noted, let's have a look at some of the only data available examining the effect of low- or no-histamine diets on Long Covid symptoms. In one of my patient-led studies (consisting of 812 long haulers), I looked at the effect on symptoms of several different groups, who in the previous month had:

- started taking supplements (non-specific)
- moved to a low- or no-histamine diet
- not changed anything (our control group).[10]

No significant improvements were noted in the supplements group, but the group who moved to a low- or no-histamine diet felt much better than the control group. The p value for the comparison of this diet change group to the control group was 0.0001.* So, it's fair to say that moving to a low- or no-histamine diet could improve symptoms. But why?

Given the potential role of MCAS in Long Covid symptoms, a potential explanation for the observed effects is that, by reducing our intake of histamine, we thereby reduce the amount our bodies have to process and don't add to the burden of the dysfunctional mast cells. Histamine intolerance can manifest in many ways that are consistent with Long Covid symptoms, such as:

- headaches or migraines
- fatigue
- hives, skin inflammation or eczema
- digestive issues
- menstrual irregularities
- nausea
- dizziness
- anxiety
- irregular heart rate.

These were the symptoms that the long haulers in my sample felt had improved after they moved to a low-histamine diet. A low-histamine diet (and, to a lesser extent, the related anti-inflammatory diet) is difficult to follow rigorously, but there are some general

---

* In statistics, the p value is a measure used to indicate the likelihood that an experimentally recorded difference between two or more groups – usually the group in which you're testing your new treatment or intervention and a control group – is due to chance. Usually, a p value boundary of 0.05 is used. If the p value for the difference between your groups is less than 0.05, then the difference is described as 'statistically significant', which means that it is unlikely to be due to chance alone. The lower the p value is beneath this threshold, the less likely it is that the observed difference between the groups is due to chance.

rules, which can make a big difference by themselves, and some excellent online resources. As the name suggests, the diet recommends avoiding the foods and substances that are either high in histamine or that deactivate the enzyme diamine oxidase in the gut, which processes histamine (and as a consequence can result in high histamine levels). You'll probably notice that on this hit list of problem foods are many of the things that give you pleasure (forming an eclectic and seemingly disconnected list) – the low-histamine diet isn't known for making its followers the life of the party:

- spicy food
- processed food
- leftovers (especially fish and meat)
- alcohol
- caffeine
- fermented food (including cheese)
- pizza
- tomatoes
- oranges
- aged or dried meat (including ham, sausages, salami and bacon)
- any fish that isn't eaten or frozen immediately on catching
- nuts
- vinegar
- soy sauce
- mustard.

A low-histamine diet makes finding food when travelling difficult and when you consider that (anecdotally) many long haulers seem to have an intolerance to gluten, the options shrink further. The general rule is to buy fresh and cook yourself (or in your household, if you don't cook it yourself) and to not eat too many leftovers if you can help it (proponents of this school of thought argue that histamine levels in many cooked foods build up over time).

In addition, if you had even a mild food or drink intolerance before you developed Long Covid, there's a chance that it has since worsened. So, if you were previously even slightly intolerant of gluten, dairy or salicylates, then I recommend cutting them out of your diet for a short period to see if it provides some relief in symptoms. Many long haulers may find that they're now intolerant to foods they previously had no issues with at all. I am now firmly in that camp, and it makes me a nightmare to cater for.

In summary, do not overlook diet. I believe it is one of the easiest things to change that can have the largest impact on your quality of life when dealing with Long Covid.

5. Stress

It is well established that stress can exacerbate diabetes and heart problems,[11, 12] but no one suggests that either of these conditions is simply a manifestation of chronic stress. Physical, mental and emotional stress all have a physiological impact on the entire body, affecting the musculoskeletal, respiratory, cardiovascular, endocrine, gastrointestinal, nervous and reproductive systems.[13] So, it's of little surprise that stress can have massive ramifications in a condition that is multi-system in nature.

Stress also affects the autonomic function of the central nervous system, thereby potentially compounding the effects of Long Covid. When the body is stressed, the sympathetic nervous system is activated into fight-or-flight mode, a state that long haulers may already be in, due to the persistent effects of the condition. The polyvagal theory (discussed in chapter 2) suggests the next stage is to tip the body into 'immobilisation', but either way what's commonly known as 'a crash' is coming.

Why do long haulers find that stress exacerbates their symptoms?
There is quite a large medical literature on the interplay between stressors, the neuroendocrine axis (the mechanism by which your nerves affect hormone release) and immune

regulation, whether in the context of inflammation, susceptibility to infection or autoimmunity. It has become the central theme of a specialist branch of immunology with its own specialist journals – the field of psychoneuroimmunology, which I've been interested in since the beginning of my research career. I started my training by considering the immune control of herpesvirus latency and reactivation, a topic explored elsewhere in this book, especially in the context of EBV. It's a given that the virus exists in the body in a state of latency (think of this as a kind of controlled hibernation) but can re-emerge in a state of full reactivation, which is often correlated with times of enhanced stress. In the field of autoimmune disease, stress has always featured high on the list of factors that can trigger a full-blown MS relapse.

Stress activates the hypothalamic–pituitary–adrenal axis and/or the sympathetic nervous system – this is part of the fight-or-flight response. Stimulation of the adrenal gland directly impacts white blood cells, including T cells, B cells and natural killer cells, changing how they produce pro-inflammatory cytokines (for example). Going back to the example of herpesvirus reactivation, a direct relationship has been demonstrated between neuroendocrine activity, immunity and viral reactivation. In studies of EBV-positive medical students, exam stress is associated with decreased ability of their T cells to kill EBV-infected cells.[14]

Stress in relation to autoimmunity has been investigated not only in terms of the risk that stress could exacerbate symptoms or trigger a relapse, but also in terms of the chance of developing the disease in the first place. In general, autoimmune diseases are considered to have genetic and environmental causes (i.e. they are caused by a combination of nature and nurture). So, for diseases like MS or type 1 diabetes, people might have specific genetic risk variants that increase their chances of getting the condition, but having the risk variants might account for less than half the overall risk of getting ill. The other share, the triggers, come from the environment. One aspect of the environment has already been discussed in this book, the internal microbiome. Among many other environmental differences between people are their infectious disease history, diet, exposure to sunlight – and levels of stress.

The issue of stress as a trigger for autoimmunity was considered in a large study looking at retrospective health records in Sweden for the period from 1981 to 2013.[15] The team used health registry records to identify more than 106,000 people who had a medical record of stress-related disorders such as acute stress reaction and post-traumatic stress disorder (PTSD). They then compared these individuals to a control group of over a million people, to determine the risk of developing any of forty-one different autoimmune diseases over a ten-year period. The answer was that the group with a clinical history of stress had a significantly enhanced risk of experiencing autoimmune diseases. However, this did not apply equally to all autoimmune diseases. It tended to affect the more endocrine presentations, for example, thyroiditis. Importantly, the risk of developing autoimmune disease was lower in people whose stress had been treated with SSRI antidepressants. In another study, which included 203,000 US army veterans with PTSD who had served in the Afghanistan or Iraq wars, a diagnosis of PTSD group was associated with a significantly raised risk of autoimmune disorders including thyroiditis, rheumatoid arthritis, MS and lupus.[16]

Your tolerance to stress while living with Long Covid is likely to be a fraction of what it used to be. The emotional stress of dealing with relationship or family issues needs only to flicker into existence and you might notice your symptoms worsening. If you're unfortunate enough to have a big fight with someone close to you, it might well lead to an equally big relapse.

Had a particularly stressful day dealing with work, but done no more physically or cognitively than any other day in the week? That is almost certainly why your post-exertional malaise has kicked in hard. If you know you're going to have a stressful day, then allocate some spoons just to the stress alone. If you get ambushed by stressful events during the day, then seriously consider dropping something from your to-do list. Trying to juggle the same number of tasks as you used to will also have negative effects. This book has already been clear about the risks of exercise (see chapter 7), so it goes without saying that physical stress is to be avoided if at all possible.

Life can be difficult and stressful as a matter of course, but there are a few things that you can do to try to minimise the burden. Talk to the people in your support network, and ask for help with the tasks you find most stressful – even if they don't take a lot of time or aren't particularly challenging. Even if the task itself doesn't require much energy, the commensurate stress level can be just as draining. If you have to do something awful like move house, hire movers if you can afford it or enlist help from family, friends or local volunteers. Many long haulers find lifting things (especially over their heads) very challenging, so moving house is one of things to avoid if at all possible if you have Long Covid.

Emotional stress often can't be avoided. If there are people in your social, work or even family circles who have a habit of winding you up, consider how much those people need to be part of your daily life and minimise your interaction with them when possible. One losing battle is trying to persuade people who don't believe you when you say that you really are sick. You may want to think about how important these people are in your life. Perhaps you could try to gently step away and let them be content in their beliefs, as difficult as that might be (see chapter 7 for more).

6. Breathwork and meditation

There is evidence that, even when breathing at a normal rate, people with Long Covid have low end-tidal carbon dioxide levels (i.e. at the end of exhaled breaths), which is also associated with PoTS.[17] Low end-tidal carbon dioxide is normally associated with hyperventilation (short or shallow breaths), and it is most likely as a consequence of sympathetic nervous system overdrive (i.e. being stuck in fight-or-flight mode).

Breathwork is a powerful tool that can help to manage your autonomic system.[18] To gain a little more insight into this area of practice, I spoke to respiratory consultant (and long hauler) Dr Asad Khan. He pointed out that breathwork and meditation are almost entirely overlooked as interventions by the Western medical system, and that as a result there is no understanding of their effectiveness as part of standard medical training. Dr Khan sees breathwork not as a woo-woo exercise to connect with your inner being, but as a way to physiologically manipulate abnormal carbon dioxide levels in your blood.

In very simple terms, breathwork can help reset this breathing imbalance and calm down the sympathetic nervous system. So, how do you do it? There are a few methods:

- coherence breathing involves inhaling for five seconds, then exhaling for five seconds (and repeat)
- box breathing involves inhaling for four seconds, holding it for four seconds, exhaling for four seconds and then waiting for four seconds before you inhale again
- the 4–7–8 breathing technique is based on a yoga technique called pranayama and unsurprisingly, as the name suggests, involves inhaling for four seconds, holding for seven seconds and then exhaling for eight seconds.

All three methods should be followed for five to ten minutes, if you can manage it. You can do any of these breathing techniques at any time. They can be particularly useful during travelling or other times you're unable to stop and rest, though it's generally recommended to sit supported or lie down on your back. Inhale through your nose and exhale through your mouth. I find that building ten minutes of breathing practice into my day at regular intervals does a remarkable job at helping me pace my way through while avoiding post-exertional malaise. US celebrity doctor Dr Andrew Weil recommends 4–7–8 breathing to aid the process of falling asleep, so it may be particularly good as an unwinding exercise.

Breathwork is an absolutely key tool to help me manage my symptoms. If I have a day when I'm unable to do it, my heart rate runs faster (objectively measured by the daily average on my Garmin watch) and the odds of me suffering post-exertional malaise the following day, for any given level of activity, are much higher.

So far, I have discussed only the usefulness of breathwork when done alone. When done one-on-one or as part of a group led by a practitioner, the effects are very different and can aid emotional release, which may also have benefits for the autonomic system – more on that in chapter 11.

What about meditation? Dr Khan argues that it works in a similar way to breathwork, only with the added benefit of minimising stimuli. By focusing on only one element – whether it's the contact of your body with the surface you're sitting on, or the breath itself – you reduce the stimuli your brain has to process and your overall allostatic load (the cumulative burden of chronic stress and life events, which, let's face it, is pretty high in Long Covid).

If you struggle with high-stimulation environments (whether visual or auditory), meditation might be up your street. Don't worry if you struggle to do it by yourself – guided meditation apps are two a penny. Big hitters like Headspace, Calm and Insight Timer are excellent.

7. Management of dysautonomia and PoTS

As we saw in chapter 2, some degree of dysautonomia seems to be present in almost all long haulers. Prof. Delaney says that in his GP practice almost every patient he's seen with Long Covid has displayed some degree of tachycardia in a simple sit-to-stand test. For those at the mild end of the spectrum, they may not be aware of the correlation between their activity and dysautonomic symptoms, whereas others who frequently experience racing heart rate, sweating, nausea and dizziness will find it plays a huge role in their daily lives.

A simple set of conservative measures can be taken to minimise dysautonomic symptoms (they also generally serve the purpose of supporting blood pressure control, which can frequently drop too low when upright):

- increase fluid intake to three or four litres of water a day
- if it is safe for you to do so, increase salt intake* (a teaspoon of salt twice daily)
- wear compression stockings or tights (ideally medical grade 2 or 3), which compensate for blood vessels in the legs not constricting and squeezing blood back into the torso
- wear an abdominal binder (as tight as you can tolerate), which also helps to control blood pressure, or a compression vest (buy one size smaller than your normal), which helps in a similar manner
- do breathwork at regular intervals
- don't be afraid to ask for disability assistance if you need to travel
- spend as much time off your feet as possible, modifying your activities if necessary to avoid time standing or walking
- try autonomic conditioning exercises (mostly performed reclining), but extreme care should be taken to avoid post-exertional malaise
- talk to your GP about the range of medications that can make a big difference (see advice in chapter 10).

8. Treatment

In the process of researching this chapter, I asked long haulers which *treatments* had made the biggest difference for them. One of

---

* If you have any pre-existing conditions, please speak to your doctor first.

the most popular responses was that the chapter should consist of a blank page. I got the gag – in that it was mostly referring to what the NHS could offer – but the reality is that there are now a number of treatments that can address symptoms effectively.

It's true that we don't yet have a proven treatment that can resolve Long Covid altogether, but if we can mitigate a number of symptoms then it could make a large difference to quality of life. In the next chapter we'll break down a vast range of treatments that long haulers have tried – from the pharmacological to the 'hands on' – and look at the evidence base for each.

GEZ: In your opinion, what are the three most important tips shared in this chapter?

DANNY: This is the chapter where you're resolutely the expert, both from all your interviews and research and from your lived experience. In this context, I'm a bit of a Luddite, sitting on the sidelines. A lot of medicine is just empirical – trying things to figure out what works and what doesn't. On that basis, I'd put the notion of rest and not trying to use exercise programmes to push your way through Long Covid near the top of the list.

As you'd expect me to say, right at the top is achieving and maintaining the highest possible level of SARS-CoV-2 immunity through vaccination and boosters. Avoiding reinfection is the most effective treatment.

GEZ: How many of these tips apply to managing other post-viral conditions, or ME/CFS for example?

DANNY: I'm very far from daring to claim any expertise in ME/CFS. I did spot that almost everything that you've been picking up on your own personal journey is very reminiscent of the ME/CFS casebook of the past several years. As we've discussed in this book, there are similarities between the described experiences of Long

Covid and ME/CFS, and people with ME/CFS can often feel slighted that their own accumulated lived experience hasn't been taken sufficiently seriously.

Summary

Depending on your particular blend of symptoms, the tips in this chapter have the potential to substantially improve your quality of life. A degree of reframing your normal expectations of what it means to live healthily is necessary, especially when it comes to notions of activity and exercise. Although almost everyone with Long Covid has their own unique experience, exercise intolerance is almost the defining attribute of the illness, and that is why *doing less* becomes an edict rather than 'take it or leave it' advice.

This chapter contains perhaps the most distinct disagreement yet (on the subject of MCAS and the benefits of low or no histamine diets) between this patient advocate and Danny's voice as a Professor of Immunology. Thankfully, much research is underway and such disputes can in time be resolved.

In the next chapter we will address the current treatment landscape, and the reasons why your doctor isn't able to give you a magic pill – yet.

CHAPTER 10: *What about Treatment?*

It's quite possible you opened this book and skipped straight to this chapter. If that's the case, I wouldn't blame you! However, there's not yet a magic pill that cures Long Covid (as opposed to practices that one can adopt to manage the condition, which we discussed in the previous chapter). In fact, the very subject of 'treatment' is so controversial that the way we address the topic in this chapter will be a little different. First Danny will speak about the subject as a whole – specifically from his perspective as a Professor of Immunology at one of the world's leading academic institutions. I will then review some of the available studies to date (notably none have yet been published in high-profile journals) and discuss the experiences of the patients who take matters into their own hands.

> **How challenging is it to address the subject of treatment for Long Covid at this time?**
> For the most part, our coming together as a double-act – a professional immunologist and a highly-informed, curious Long Covid patient, film-maker and communicator – has been a joy. We've bounced ideas off each other and, I think, both learnt from each other. As will become apparent, the banter became a little less smooth and easy-going when it came to any agreement on how to present the outlook for treatments. Later in this chapter, Gez writes about his personal journey as a long hauler, impatient for help and prepared to take some personal risks – essentially acting as a human guinea pig. I have to say that I read his first draft and was shocked: I can't recommend or endorse untried, unlicensed, non-evidenced and – sometimes

– potentially dangerous treatments. My aim in presenting this polarisation is simply to point out that with a new, common disease process that has so suddenly come to the fore and for which the agenda is being driven forward by patients rather than the medical establishment, we find ourselves in difficult, uncharted territory. We need to have some new, difficult discussions and, maybe, establish some new, faster ways of doing things – just as how we'd imagined that developing new vaccines took decades, until in the heat of battle we needed them in less than a year. If this book can help to trigger some of those policy discussions about faster routes to trial and licensing, that would be a job well done.

On a personal level, I'm rather attached to a modus operandi based on rigorously evidenced treatments that have run the gauntlet of professional approval for efficacy. This tends to involve huge controlled clinical trials that produce unequivocal evidence with great p values (a measure of the probability that a treatment's effects are not due to chance) such that the cost–benefit of rolling out this treatment would be undeniable. In the UK, this would involve approval by NICE. It is hard to emphasise sufficiently the critical importance of carefully designed and statistically powered randomised controlled trials in establishing efficacy, and the confounder posed both by placebo effects and by simply chasing after 'hunches' from inconclusive trials. Clearly there may be a trade-off calculation that clinicians need to do until good data arrives. There may be a lower threshold for established medicines with known side-effect profiles, and no or incredibly rare potentially serious side effects (think antihistamines, for example); and a higher threshold for when there is less clear safety data or there are known and significant potential harms. All of this must be balanced against the severity/chronicity of the individual's illness: two-years of symptoms with great distress, loss of function and with no sign of natural recovery may be very different in terms of calculating potential benefits (and the cost of just doing nothing) to six months of symptoms, still able to function and showing some signs of things going in the right direction in terms of recovery. Set against this backdrop, I get worried when I see that desperate patients are paying sometimes huge and unaffordable sums of money to private practitioners, at home or abroad, for treatments that haven't yet crossed this line. I accept that, in some cases, this may simply mean that the process is too slow, and they feel forced to pay to take a chance on the fast-track to a possible answer. In other cases, I'm afraid, I see exploitation of scared and vulnerable people by those offering snake oil 'solutions' and tests at exploitative costs – approaches that will never cross the efficacy line. I also worry about the personal dangers to health posed by some non-trivial interventions, and the sheer confusion and delay caused by conflating personal anecdotes and statistically powered trials.

I've worked on many diseases in my career. In every case, whether thinking about unknowns in MS, type 1 diabetes or bacterial sepsis, there was a background of many thousands of publications and decades, often centuries, of research. The issue was to spot the murky, poorly described parts of the narrative, full molecular descriptions of which would facilitate entirely new approaches. Thus, the role of the incoming researcher was to spot these unknowns, formulate a hypothesis that might be addressed with a new approach and, if able to convince funders of the potential of this knowledge increment, nudge the field forward just a little.

The process has sometimes felt glacial, but the period I've spent in immunology has been a joy in terms of seeing great laboratory science bear fruit and change people's everyday lives with revolutionary treatments. When I was a PhD student and then a post-doc researcher, articles would end optimistically with crystal-ball gazing about how the immunological insights discussed therein would one day pave the way for finely tuned treatments based on immune modulation. Now I'm (a little) older and greyer, and these life-changing treatments are routine in clinics all around me. They are based on precisely the promises from those earlier papers. There's now an arsenal of different monoclonal antibodies (manufactured antibodies countering the effect of an inflammatory protein) for people with rheumatoid arthritis or inflammatory bowel disease or MS, which do everything from blocking inflammatory cytokines to depleting B cells or blocking traffic of T cells into the central nervous system.

I spent a large part of my career at what was then called the Imperial Cancer Research Fund, the major cancer research institute in the UK. When those of us in immunology research programmes (not the most popular in the building) would give our weekly seminars on how immune cells can kill tumours and that one day this would become the basis for effective treatments, we faced disbelief from much of the audience. Today, so-called 'immunotherapy', which takes the brakes off T cells, allowing for better tumour killing, is an effective first port of call in many cancer treatment regimens. Immunology research can achieve amazing things – but it takes time. My dispute with what Gez outlines in the remainder of this chapter is about the specific route and timescale to get to that point.

As new treatments are trialled, published, licensed and adopted into protocols, consensus international treatment guidelines are agreed, redrafted, peer reviewed and published. This is how treatments make their slow and winding journey from the laboratory to the bedside. In the twenty-first century, the practice of medicine is guided by protocols and consensus guidelines, which often offer a clear flow-chart detailing which drugs to give and when. There's little space for the maverick to follow their hunches and try something off-piste. Such actions could potentially lead to adverse outcomes, patient complaints and legal cases. Modern medicine is rightly cautious and conservative. Even minor deviations from tried-and-tested protocols are often the subject of intense debate at 'multi-disciplinary team meetings' about minimising patient risks. The decision is very much a collective one.

To many of those with Long Covid who are counting the days until they can get their former lives back, the old arguments for slow and steady conservatism will rankle. On social media, I see a torrent of comments pushing for one or another treatment (or an expensive private assay or test) to be made widely available and tested immediately. Mixed in with the despair, irritation and anger, one often senses a degree of conspiracy theory: they – that is, the government or the medical establishment – know this new treatment is obviously the answer, so what factors could possibly be making them withhold the treatment from us?

At this stage, it is worth looking at the timeline of the RECOVERY trial – the UK-funded programme to fast-track randomised controlled trials (RCTs) of treatments for acute Covid (it's particularly apposite to do so as many are lobbying for the 'RECOVERY trial for Long Covid' – hard to argue with). RECOVERY was conceived during the early days of pandemic horror, when many potential treatments were posited, including chloroquine, ivermectin and, more conventionally, transfer of convalescent plasma (i.e. plasma donated by people who had had Covid and recovered).

RECOVERY involved hundreds of doctors and tens of thousands of patients across 198 large NHS hospitals, and aimed to drive huge statistically powered RCTs. The draft protocol was written by 10 March 2020 – that is, at a time when alarm was rising but the UK had yet to go into lockdown. Ethics was granted and within a few months thousands of hospitalised patients had entered the trial. Powerful, credible results emerged fairly rapidly and were published in the top-notch, peer-reviewed medical journals. Some approaches that had seemed like a good bet offered no benefit at all, while others were statistically confirmed to have real clinical benefit. For all treatments that were trialled in RECOVERY, there were strong suggestions of benefits in smaller trials. However, treatments like hydroxychloroquine, aspirin, convalescent plasma, azithromycin (an antibiotic often used for its anti-inflammatory benefits in the lung) and lopinavir–ritonavir (a combination antiviral developed for treatment of HIV) proved ineffective in the trial. Other treatments produced proven benefits – most importantly perhaps the corticosteroid dexamethasone, which cut deaths by about a third.

It should be immediately apparent that there is a difference between the terms of reference for the original RECOVERY trial, which was aimed at treating acute cases of Covid in hospitalised patients, and a potential corresponding trial for Long Covid. In the former case, there was a clear, agreed premise that people were dying from a new presentation of viral pneumonia. Thus, the top candidate treatments were those that already had the strongest track-record either for blocking the virus or for stopping excessive or inappropriate lung inflammation. But where do we start in drawing up the equivalent top candidates for trial in Long Covid, when we lack any consensus on the cause or stratification of the disease? How do we design drug trials that might accommodate and group together the people with brain fog, tinnitus, tachycardia and dizziness, and also those with shortness of breath, fatigue and fevers? What about all the hundreds of patterns in between and patients whose disease profile is relapsing and remitting or evolving? Before we leave RECOVERY, it's worth noting that lots of high-granularity data was collected for the primary outcome of severity of, and survival from, acute infection. There would be great value in revisiting this data to look at the longer-term outcomes for risk of Long Covid. The answers may be different – that is, we may get positive answers for additional drug approaches – and this could be valuable for reducing future cases.

I conducted a rather non-scientific straw-poll of colleagues running Long Covid clinics, asking them to name, off the top of their heads, the most commonly prescribed drugs there? The initial answer was often that their role was more to refer patients on to the specific clinical specialty where they could get specialist tests and therapeutics – such as neurology, respiratory medicine or cardiology. The drugs most frequently mentioned were antihistamines, colchicine, amitriptyline and, more rarely, heparin as an anticoagulant. Colchicine (which had no effect on acute Covid in the RECOVERY trial) has most commonly been used as a treatment for inflammation in gout, but has anti-inflammatory effects in the lung. Amitriptyline used to be given as an antidepressant but is now more often used in pain syndromes, including fibromyalgia, migraine and tension headaches. Some colleagues are prescribing ivabradine for the significant proportion with PoTs.

What about looking a little further into the future? There are currently some outstanding studies underway around the world to look at the pathogenesis of Long Covid. If these start to provide some consensus answers, perhaps over the next year, they could lead in exciting directions in terms of treatment options. As we discussed in chapter 4, there are several, non-mutually exclusive working hypotheses for the mechanisms underpinning Long Covid. Viewed in this light, there are clearly many different types of therapeutics that will need to be considered, ranked and trialled; some are readily available and relatively low-risk, such as the antihistamines that form one arm of the STIMULATE-ICP trial led by University College London.

Given the promising but still equivocal evidence that Covid vaccination can alleviate Long Covid symptoms in at least some patients, there will be obvious interest in trials that investigate therapies that target possible viral reservoirs, such as antivirals and neutralising monoclonal antibodies. For my taste, this is the low-hanging fruit in the search for quick wins in Long Covid, if only we can become better at identifying those with real evidence of persistent infection. Other candidate treatments are somewhat higher-risk and non-trivial, such as anticoagulation therapy, which is associated with risks of bleeds into the brain or gut. If we end up going down the road of immunotherapy to modulate immune subsets, there will be exciting prospects for finely tuned answers. However, the immune system operates in a very fine balance, with every subset there for a good evolutionary reason. Thus, any depletion comes with potential costs.

I can almost hear the approaching Twitterstorm of fury from those who feel they have already waited too long and would rather take the plunge and just try things. My position is that, if done well, as in RECOVERY, trials can very rapidly progress to solutions that offer tangible benefit (and those that are not useful can be crossed off the list). Personal experiments with a sample size of one patient will never shift us out of this horrific crisis or have any hope of discovering which treatments work. Instead, we should start policy dialogue about how to invest in huge trials that can find some big, compelling answers.

The literature

One of the challenges of a novel condition that affects so many people all around the world is the demands it puts on our system of evidence-based medicine. The need for rigorous evidence is what differentiates modern medicine from the quacks and snake oil merchants of the past. Danny is of course correct when he demands that the standards to which we hold our evidence cannot be compromised, especially when the wellbeing of so many people is at stake. Do we want to deal with Long Covid the same way the medical establishment dealt with the 'hysteria' of ME/CFS (before the condition even had a name)? Of course not. However, the problem remains when a new condition arrives: how do you build up the research evidence in a way that can be relied upon? Right now, we have a few small studies. The results from some of these may well be replicated later by large, well-designed randomised controlled trials (RCTs). Other promising-looking studies may offer results that later turn out to be a bust. This is the stage the research is currently at for Long Covid – a few small studies but nothing even close to definitive yet. We are still waiting on those large RCTs.

So, if we look at the studies that *have* been published so far, how do we separate 'trustworthy' evidence from poor evidence? How are we to tell a good trial from a bad trial? One of the tools we have is the hierarchy-of-evidence pyramid, which conveys how much stock we should take in any given treatment. The gold standard of evidence is the RCT, but at the time of writing only one RCT of a treatment for Long Covid has been published. The next step level on the pyramid are large cohort studies, but we don't have any of these yet. We have to go down another level to case-control studies, in which one group is given a treatment and another matched group is used as a control. The groups generally aren't blinded – that is to say, the control group and treatment group both know which group they're in, and placebos aren't given.

The next level of evidence we'll turn to are published case series, smaller studies that don't include any control group and in which all participants know that they are receiving the treatment (unlike a blinded trial). After that, the next tier of evidence we'll turn to are preprints, which almost exist in a parallel pyramid of their own. Preprints are research papers that have yet to be peer reviewed or accepted by a journal. The quality of preprints can be wildly variable, because anyone can write a paper and publish it on a preprint server.

The following level of evidence we'll consider is patient-led data, such as my own. While the sample sizes in my data are often larger than some of the clinical studies to date, this data is subject to selection and reporting biases. Finally, we'll take a look at by far the largest tier – the one at the bottom, below even the editorials and expert opinion shown in the diagram – anecdotal evidence.

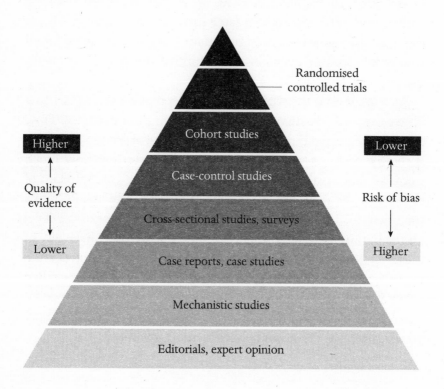

Long Covid is such a new condition, and it takes so long to do sophisticated research (including gaining funding, getting ethics approval, recruiting patients, actually doing the study, analysing the data and publishing the findings), that it is inevitable that most treatment will still be at the anecdotal stage. Some of these treatments may have evidence for efficacy in other conditions, but their use in Long Covid is 'off-label'; other treatments are holistic in nature and are unlikely to ever get tested in RCTs. For this anecdotal tier, we will look at the science that backs up the treatment idea itself, what the risks might be and ultimately whether there might be anything to it.

It's also important to note that not all RCTs are created equal: there is a huge difference between an RCT published in a top journal and a small one. A well-designed large case-control study published in a prestigious journal may well constitute far better evidence than a small RCT that is published in a little-known journal (which may have less stringent standards in terms of the quality of evidence and peer review). The impact factor is a calculation that reflects the total number of papers published by a journal versus the number of times its papers have been cited (the more citations relative to number of papers, the more 'impactful' the journal). The world's leading journals, such as *Science, Nature, The Lancet, The New England Journal of Medicine* and *Cell* have impact factors of between forty-one and ninety-two, while other respectable journals might have scores of between five and ten, and journals that are rarely read or cited might have scores of one or less. Right now, as Danny alluded to, we don't have any studies published in the world's leading journals, so that context is important. I will state the impact factor (per 2021 figures) for the journals that the following studies are published in. Of course, it is perfectly possible for excellent science to be published in less well-established journals, so don't take the impact factor of a journal as an absolute indicator of quality!

As Danny says, long haulers have been so desperate for treatment that, over the past two or three years, they have tried just about everything. If I've heard about it, then it's included in my anecdotal list, which is as comprehensive as we have space for in the book. I must stress that you should talk to your GP before starting any new treatment, as there may be complex interactions with existing medication that may not be immediately apparent, as well as other possible risks.

This is also a fast-moving landscape: some treatments that are currently in the anecdotal tier may move up as trials get conducted and papers published, while others that are currently on the pyramid may come down or off altogether as contrary evidence emerges. This is the nature of science and ever-evolving research into a new condition. Writing this chapter is akin to building a castle on the beach as the tide is coming. So, with that disclaimer out of the way, let's dive in.

RCTs

If there was one RCT that the community would love to see take place sooner rather than later, it would be a trial of Paxlovid – a combination medication consisting of the antivirals nirmatrelvir and ritonavir that is often prescribed to people hospitalised with acute Covid. If viral persistence in immune privileged reservoirs (as discussed in chapter 4) is causing Long Covid, Paxlovid could be effective in wiping these reservoirs out. However, at the time of writing, an RCT of Paxlovid in Long Covid looks a long way off, so we have to make do with the only RCT that has been done in Long Covid, which looked at probiotics.

The UK Phyto-V study was published in the journal *COVID* (no impact factor available, due to the newness of the journal), and looked at the efficacy of a phytochemical-rich food capsule at moderating symptoms compared with placebo in 147 patients with either acute or Long Covid.[1] The findings suggested that intake of the capsule (in addition to a pre- and probiotic capsule, which all patients in the trial took) statistically improved self-reported symptoms including fatigue and cough, as well as general wellbeing. It should be noted, though, that improvements in fatigue were recorded on the Chalder Fatigue Scale, which has come under criticism in some quarters for not being able to accurately measure the extent of the problem in ME/CFS.

Gut health has long been a subject of interest in the Long Covid community, so to many of us this finding has not been a huge surprise. There are also evidence-based approaches built from an assumption that inflammatory disease can ensue from dysbiosis – i.e. unfavourable alteration of the bacterial make-up of the gut microbiome. Probiotics can help to correct this dysbiosis, decreasing gut inflammation and improving gut wall integrity.[2,3] One team in Hong Kong considers the association between microbiota species and Long Covid sufficiently strong to have developed a Long Covid predictive test on this basis.[4] This is a subject to be watched with great interest going forwards.

There are several other RCTs underway of other Long Covid treatments, which we will address in the next chapter.

Cohort studies

As far as we're aware, at the time of writing no cohort studies have yet been published (due to the paucity of published research generally). So, the state of play in this tier of the pyramid is very much: 'Move along, nothing to see here.'

Case-control studies

Published case-control studies are also rather thin on the ground, but positive results have been published for two treatments: antihistamines and sulodexide.

ANTIHISTAMINES

In an open label (where both the health providers and patients are aware of the treatment being given) observational study published in the *Journal of Investigative Medicine* (which is part of the *British Medical Journal Group* and has an impact factor of 2.9), a group of twenty-six long haulers took a combination of either loratadine or fexofenadine (which block H1 histamine receptors) and famotidine or nizatidine (which block H2 histamine receptors) and were compared with another group of twenty-three long haulers who did not take them (the trial also included a group of sixteen people who had recovered uneventfully from acute Covid).[5] Patients taking antihistamines reported gradual improvement in all symptoms (although the authors didn't compare changes in symptoms between groups) except dysautonomia, suggesting that dysautonomic symptoms arise through a different mechanism. The authors proposed that the antihistamines could function as T-cell modulators, given T-cell function was observed to be perturbed across the sample of long haulers. Limitations of this study include the open label nature – where the placebo effect could play a part in any observed changes. Also the patients were not randomised, so there may be differences between the treated and un-treated groups that could explain the different outcomes.

In chapter 1 we discussed the possible phenotypes of Long Covid. For those who identify with MCAS symptoms (especially with any kind of allergy), this treatment could be particularly helpful. Anecdotally, antihistamines are critical to my management of the condition. For me they help control skin inflammation, and if I'm even half an hour later than usual with my evening dose, I can already feel my skin getting hot and itchy. I haven't been off them for long enough to see which of my other symptoms they might also help mitigate.

Some of the antihistamines used in the study were prescription medications, but over-the-counter antihistamines are available. Dr Tina Peers (who has a special interest in MCAS) also recommends antihistamines widely for treating Long Covid, and suggests trying different over-the-counter brands to see which work best for you – everyone is a little different.[6] Even if you decide to take over-the-counter antihistamines, it is still worth discussing this choice with your doctor first to rule out any contraindications or other risk factors.

SULODEXIDE

I'm not aware of anyone who has been prescribed sulodexide for Long Covid, but a conference abstract published in the *Archives of*

Cardiovascular Diseases (impact factor 2.3) investigated its use in the condition.[7] Sulodexide is normally used for preventing and treating thromboembolic diseases (when clots travel through the vascular system and can get lodged in inappropriate places with awful results), so given the vascular nature of Long Covid its use does make some sense.

In the study, seventy-nine patients received sulodexide treatment, and twenty-one days later the treated group presented with less severe Long Covid symptoms, including chest pain, palpitations, fatigue and neurocognitive difficulties, than those who had not received the treatment. The authors conclude that sulodexide may be a good intervention in patients with endothelial dysfunction who are experiencing these symptoms. However, more studies will need to replicate these results before this becomes a widely used treatment.

Case series

There are only two published case series in Long Covid to our knowledge, one involving hyperbaric oxygen therapy and one of stellate ganglion blocking.

HYPERBARIC OXYGEN THERAPY

Hyperbaric oxygen therapy is an established treatment for carbon monoxide poisoning, gangrene and stubborn wounds. It involves going into a tank in which the atmospheric pressure is raised and there is much more oxygen than in standard air, which causes which you to breathe in more oxygen. It seems to be beneficial in people with problems with gas exchange (getting your tissues to process the oxygen and return carbon dioxide to the blood) or hypoperfusion (where the tissues don't get enough oxygen).

In a small UK case series published in *Clinical Medicine* (impact factor 2.7), ten patients received ten sessions each of hyperbaric oxygen therapy (at 2.4 atmospheres of pressure) over a twelve-day period.[8] The trial found that the treatment resulted in a statistically significant improvement in fatigue, cognition, executive function, information processing and verbal function. Some questions remain, though, especially given that the placebo effect is likely quite strong given the immersive nature of treatment, and the scepticism with which HBOT is regarded as a treatment by the medical establishment (outside of specific complaints such as carbon monoxide poisoning or 'the bends'). How long-lasting are the benefits? Given the significant expense, how many sessions at what pressure are required to see improvement? Hyperbaric oxygen chambers capable of running these pressures are also incredibly thin on the ground, so access is difficult. The chambers found in 'wellness' clinics are more numerous, but run at lower pressures and we don't yet have any data of the benefits at those lower pressures.

I tried several series of hyperbaric oxygen therapy at a lower pressure and found that they substantially improved my cognitive dysfunction, alertness and energy levels, and reduced headaches and post-exertional malaise. However, after a week or two the benefit would slip away if I wasn't continuing with regular treatments. It seems (from my experience and that of others I've spoken to) that unless you can deal with the underlying pathology, hyperbaric oxygen therapy isn't resolving the problem itself – it is simply squirting some nitrous into your tank for a temporary boost (for those *Fast and Furious* fans out there).

STELLATE GANGLION BLOCK

This rare procedure involves an anaesthetic injection to a specific area in the neck where your sympathetic nerves run to other parts of your body. It has been used to treat PTSD, Complex Regional Pain Syndrome, and has been hypothesised to have a potential role in Long Covid. A paper in the *Journal of Neuroimmunology* (impact factor 3.5) details the use of the treatment in two patients with Long Covid, with a view to blocking the sympathetic nervous system and allowing the regional autonomic nervous system to 'reboot'.[9]

The study found that symptoms as wide-ranging as fatigue, cough, chest pain, headache, dizziness and post-exertional malaise all improved (and remained improved two months after treatment). However, this is a very small study where the placebo effect would be sizeable, so it would be good to see these findings replicated in further research.

Preprints

There are many preprint studies out there of a wide range of treatments in patients with Long Covid. I have focused here on those that have found huge traction in the community. It's worth noting again that preprints have not yet been peer reviewed, and can be published by just about anyone online, so the quality of the evidence can be widely variable (i.e. preprints can include papers that are unlikely to find a journal that would publish them *anywhere*, as well as those that will ultimately end up peer reviewed and published in a top journal). Important trials are generally fast tracked for publication so high quality preprints tend not to stay unpublished for long.

'TRIPLE ANTICOAGULANT THERAPY'

In light of the emerging evidence of microclots in the blood of long haulers (see chapter 5), a team looked at the effectiveness of treating the microclotting pathology by targeting the hyperactivated platelets potentially responsible.[10] After checking the blood of seventy long haulers – and finding microclots and platelet pathology in *all* samples – they treated twenty-four participants with a combination of three drugs – two targeting platelet function (clopidogrel and aspirin) and an anticoagulant (apixaban). Over a month, microclot levels dropped, as did the level of platelet hyperactivation, and all treated patients reported an improvement in their Long Covid symptoms.

It's worth noting that twenty-four treated patients constitutes a small study, and there was no control group to compare results with to establish whether improvements were statistically significant. The patients were not blinded, so they all knew they were receiving treatment and the placebo effect could have been significant. In addition, the problem with prescribing this medication in the UK is that there needs to be a clinical indication for use, and GP surgeries are not able to do the fluorescence microscopy required to identify microclots or hyperactivated platelets. In fact, there isn't even agreement yet among haematologists on what the structures viewed under microscopy are – microclots or something else? There are also significant risks of excessive bleeding during treatment, so informed consent regarding the risks and potential benefits, as well as careful supervision by the prescribing doctor, would be essential.

MARAVIROC AND PRAVASTATIN

In this yet to be peer-reviewed case series, eighteen long haulers who met specific inclusion criteria (elevated cytokine levels, and an absence of EBV and Lyme disease) were treated with a combination of maraviroc (an antiretroviral drug developed to treat HIV, but in this case intended to lower certain cytokine levels) and pravastatin (normally used to reduce cholesterol and prevent heart disease).[11]

After six to twelve weeks, significant clinical improvement was reported in neurological, autonomic, respiratory, cardiac and fatigue symptoms, which corresponded with significant decreases in the vascular markers sCD40L and VEGF (which have previously been associated with Long Covid severity).[12]

It's very hard to find a doctor in the UK who will prescribe maraviroc. Any prescription issued would be private, and it's an extremely expensive treatment (costing £500–1000 per month) with significant potential harms. Anecdotally, I've also seen long haulers on this treatment experience debilitating side effects. Once again, we'll need to see published RCTs on this treatment before it's likely to be widely available on this side of the Atlantic, as the evidence base is still extremely weak.

IVERMECTIN

Here's an *extremely* hot potato. Ivermectin, the drug previously best known for worming horses (and sometimes humans), burst onto the Covid scene in 2020, quickly following hydroxychloroquine as a populist choice for treating acute infection. It was mooted to have strong antiviral and ant-inflammatory properties based on in-vitro (i.e. lab-based) experiments.

In an early preprint from July 2020, thirty-three Peruvian patients with prolonged Covid symptoms were given ivermectin between four and twelve weeks after their initial infection.[13] The paper states that 88% of the patients saw total clinical improvement (i.e. all symptoms disappeared) after two doses of ivermectin, and total or partial improvement was seen in 94% of the cohort.

To our knowledge, this is the only data out there on the treatment of Long Covid with ivermectin. The results at first glance look pretty spectacular – if they are to be believed, then here's our magic bullet, right? Well, not so fast. The paper has more holes in it than Harry Styles's hideaway boat in the film *Dunkirk*, including a complete absence of any detail on objective or even subjective measurement of symptoms – either before or after treatment. There is no information on whether the improvement was sustained. The paper states nothing about the nature of the cohort, other than that all of them were still in the immediate post-viral stage of the acute infection – without accounting for the fact that many long haulers' Long Covid symptoms don't even begin until three months after initial infection.

Nevertheless, ivermectin is *notionally* a safe and relatively accessible drug that many long haulers, especially in the earlier days of Long Covid awareness, felt like it was worth taking a punt on. I know people who've said it made them feel better, and others who have said it made no difference.

I tried it myself, but with disastrous consequences. After a six-day course of ivermectin in September 2021, I was admitted to hospital with acute eosinophilia (high levels of eosinophils, a type of white blood cell), likely due to a massive reaction to the drug.

Most of my skin flaked off my body, my inguinal lymph nodes had swollen to the size of golf balls, and I was shivering constantly (known as rigors). I spent five days as a patient at the Royal Free Hospital in London, where I was treated with intravenous fluids and paracetamol. I was severely unwell. Fortunately, I recovered without lasting damage. Given this experience, I can't recommend that anyone take ivermectin for Long Covid.

This experience shows just how desperate Long Covid can make us. The combination of extremely poor quality of life, the unclear prognosis and the absence of any 'official' treatment means that long haulers (including myself at that stage) will take unknown risks if there's some chance it might help them in any way. Because at some level it feels like there's nothing to lose. However, it's never worth taking risks on medication that you're unfamiliar with if you're not under the care of a supervising doctor. Beyond simply the doctor's ability to prescribe, their role is to carefully consider the evidence for efficacy and safety, which should lead to a considered discussion of your individual circumstances and thus informed consent. I don't know anyone who's rolled the dice on a random drug and found they were suddenly cured, so don't be tempted by social media stories that say something along those lines. There is far more risk than reward.

Patient-led research

Towards the bottom of the pyramid is where things get a bit foggy. Preprints could almost exist on a separate pyramid of their own, and while patient-led research isn't necessarily any less robust or rigorous than 'official' research, it is a highly variable and unregulated arena. As a consequence, I'm conservatively placing my studies below the preprints and above the anecdotal stories.

NIACIN

In a survey of 812 long haulers in November 2020, I looked at a group of 672 who had changed their diet or started taking new supplements or medications in the last month, versus a control group

of 140 who had not.[14] I broke down those who had changed something in the last month into a few different groups:

- started supplements only (any new supplement)
- started any new supplements and medications
- adopted a low-histamine diet (with some people also
  taking supplements or niacin)
- started niacin (also known as vitamin B3) only.

Only two groups showed a statistically significant improvement in
their Long Covid symptoms when compared with the control
group: those who adopted a low-histamine diet (p=0.0001), and
those who started taking niacin (p=0.01).

Niacin seemed to improve fatigue, neurological, GI symptoms and
insomnia symptoms, whereas those who adopted a low-histamine diet
in addition to niacin improved in all categories, including breathlessness, tachycardia and anxiety – and by even larger margins in the
other symptom categories than those taking niacin only did. Of
course, I have to mention there are several limitations to this data,
from the self-reported nature of the adopted measures and subjective
improvements, to the usual issues of placebo response, the low sample
size of the low-histamine diet group, and the fact that some respondents in this group may have been taking other medications (such as
antihistamines), which might have had an effect on their symptoms.

These limitations duly noted, why does niacin seem to improve
symptoms? In chapter 5, I outlined the research suggesting that
metabolic dysfunction could be responsible for at least some Long
Covid symptoms. Niacin, in its nicotinic acid form, is a precursor of
the essential coenzyme NAD+, a deficiency of which may contribute to many of the symptom patterns we see in long haulers.

In chapter 5 we addressed the possible role of MCAS and subsequent histamine intolerance. A low-histamine diet (as described in
the previous chapter) may work to mitigate some of the pathology
that antihistamines also look to counter.

Niacin supplements are available over the counter, but higher
doses can cause an unpleasant flushing effect as a result of its

vasodilatory properties. This can be mitigated by taking a low-dose aspirin (75mg, not the standard 300mg tablets used for pain relief) at the same time or by eating an apple (the pectin in the apple skin counters this effect). Needless to say, please do talk to your doctor before starting to take niacin or any over-the-counter medication if you have any concerns at all.[15]

Symptomatic Relief

This section doesn't fit cleanly into the Long Covid evidence pyramid we've established, rather these treatments exist high up in their own adjacent pyramids, being medications that have an established evidence base for treating other conditions or symptoms. They are included here as they have been used as treatments for Long Covid or parts of its symptomatic presentation.

CORTICOSTEROIDS

This class of drugs act as an immunosuppressant and anti-inflammatories, and can be taken either in a tablet form or inhaled for breathing difficulties (like with asthma). One particular drug, dexamethasone, demonstrated efficacy in severe acute Covid in the RECOVERY trial, but another steroid – prednisolone – is more often prescribed to treat symptoms in long haulers.

Many of those who take prednisolone report an improvement in symptoms while on the drug, and it can be very effective in managing acute flares. However, high doses are only tolerated for short periods and even lower doses can have extremely significant side effects (like Cushing's syndrome) when taken long term. Given the temporary nature of improvement and the serious side effects, steroids aren't currently considered to be a first-line treatment for Long Covid. However, there is an argument for trialling steroids early in the Long Covid disease course, or even post-acute infection to see if they might help to prevent the development of the condition, but time will tell whether such research gets off the ground.

SSRIS AND ANTIDEPRESSANTS

SSRIs are usually prescribed for anxiety and depression, and work by regulating serotonin levels (a neurotransmitter connected to mood, emotion and sleep) in the body. These are usually prescribed to manage the mood disturbances common in Long Covid, as well as post-traumatic stress disorder and to a lesser degree, dizziness. Amitriptyline can be prescribed to help with headaches, pain and insomnia. Duloxetine can be prescribed to help with pain, while mirtazapine can help with sleep problems or weight loss.

PAINKILLERS

Over the counter painkillers such as paracetamol, ibuprofen and aspirin can be effective symptomatic relief for headaches or other pain, while a considered discussion with your doctor about co-codamol or opiates might be required if you are suffering particularly severely. Other (prescription) options for treating pain include gabapentin, pregabalin and lidocaine patches. TENS devices can also be effective, and are closely related to the vagal nerve stimulation devices mentioned later in this chapter.

MAST CELL MANAGEMENT

Montelukast is a drug best known to people with asthma, in whom it is prescribed to help manage shortness of breath. It prevents the release of histamine by stabilising the membrane of the mast cell itself. Montelukast is taken by some long haulers to manage symptoms connected to MCAS, although accessing it does require a very sympathetic prescriber to consider prescribing it off-label. Another drug in this category is ketotifen, which has been reported to help with sleep when taken at night.

CARDIOVASCULAR DRUGS

Beta blockers, including bisoprolol and propranolol, can often be prescribed to deal with PoTS symptoms, although they do come with some potential side effects, including fatigue, nightmares and worsening of asthma. Alternative drugs often prescribed to deal with the orthostatic hypotension (i.e. low blood pressure upon standing) of dysautonomia and PoTS include, fludrocortisone, ivabradine and midodrine. It's reasonable to ask your GP about ivabradine, but the vasoconstrictor midodrine is more of a rare beast and more commonly prescribed by specialist consultants.

COLCHICINE

Colchicine is a medication commonly used to treat gout, but some Long Covid clinics prescribe it to long haulers to help with pericarditis (swelling of the tissue around the heart). Those who've taken it have also reported some improvement in their Long Covid symptoms generally. Colchicine has anti-platelet properties, and this may be contributing to some of the improvement, given what we know about the potential roles of endotheliitis and hyper-activated platelets in Long Covid.[16] It is worth noting that Colchicine did not show efficacy against acute Covid in the RECOVERY trial.

NON-STEROIDAL ANTI-INFLAMMATORY DRUGS

This common drug class includes both aspirin and ibuprofen, both of which could be useful in Long Covid in potentially different ways. In low doses, aspirin has anti-platelet properties and could be used to counter the 'sticky blood' that many long haulers have.[17] Ibuprofen is an anti-inflammatory as well as a painkiller. Both of these drugs have risks and potential side effects, particularly when used long term, so get advice from your doctor before taking them regularly.

HORMONE REPLACEMENT THERAPY

This category also encompasses supplemental testosterone, oestrogen or progesterone. In chapter 6 Dr Tania Dempsey discussed in an interview with me how she often prescribes progesterone to help women in particular manage the hormonal swings that come with their cycle and that seem to drive flares in Long Covid symptoms. I've not heard of any men using supplemental testosterone, but the women who have been prescribed it report a generally positive experience.

Anecdotal

In this final tier of the pyramid, we will address the treatments that I have heard long haulers report improvement from, but there is currently no trial evidence or data to support their use. The sample sizes, given the anecdotal nature of the stories, is usually a handful of people, at most.

Why include these treatments in this chapter? If you are a long hauler, you are almost certain to hear others claiming incredible results with one or more of them, so I wanted to provide a factual myth-busting resource to deflate any possible miracle cures that you might see touted online or elsewhere. We will start by looking at a couple of medications that don't have the established evidence base to fit the category above, before moving onto supplements and finally taking on behavioural interventions and practices.

PAXLOVID

Paxlovid is a combination antiviral drug that is used to treat serious acute cases of Covid, where it has demonstrated 89% efficacy at reducing hospital admission and death.[18] The hypothesis supporting its usefulness in Long Covid is based on the assumption there is still viral persistence in the body driving symptoms, which the drug will help to eliminate.

The only evidence for its efficacy in Long Covid currently comes from a handful of long haulers who have claimed on social media that their symptoms have resolved after taking a course of Paxlovid for a new infection. However, I am aware of as many long haulers who have taken the drug for a similar reason but found themselves back to their normal Long Covid baseline afterwards. Some people *do* have a persistent reservoir of SARS-CoV-2 long after acute infection, but whether this is definitely correlated with persistent symptoms is unclear. If we knew for certain who had a chronic viral infection and who didn't, we'd have a better idea of who might benefit from Paxlovid or monoclonal antibody therapy – both of these are therapeutics that would be predicted to ablate any chronic viral persistence. The gold standard for looking at viral persistence is gut biopsy, but this is rarely done (or ethically sanctioned) outside of the gastroenterology clinic. It had been hoped that viral PCR of stool samples may be a non-invasive proxy, but the correlation actually seems rather poor.[19] If we could agree on a means of stratifying those individuals with clear evidence of persistent infection, a Paxlovid trial should be on the priority list.

NALTREXONE

Naltrexone is usually used to help people overcome opioid addiction, but in very low doses (under a tenth of those used to treat opioid use disorder) it can function as a painkiller and and an anti-inflammatory. Studies (from journals with impact factors between 2.3 and 3.0) have investigated the use of low-dose naltrexone in pain, fibromyalgia and ME/CFS.[20–22] There is currently a pilot study looking into the drug's efficacy in Long Covid,[23] based on a hypothesis that LDN might mediate inflammation and immune activation in the brain.[24] As a treatment, low-dose naltrexone is promising but clearly more research is needed.

MELATONIN

Melatonin is a naturally occurring hormone that governs the sleep–wake cycle. It can help with falling asleep at night, which many long haulers struggle with, despite our general state of perpetual exhaustion.

CANNABIDIOL (CBD) OIL

Some long haulers swear by CBD oil (derived from the cannabis plant, but completely legal and widely available, albeit in a very low dose in the UK), and a phase 2 trial is currently underway in the UK to test its efficacy.[25] I have tried it and found it helped with headaches, but it's relatively expensive and in my experience the benefits do not last very long.

DIAMINE OXIDASE

Diamine oxidase is an enzyme responsible for breaking down histamine in the stomach, and people who don't have enough of it often experience histamine intolerance. It stands to reason that if you're experiencing histamine intolerance (or have just had a histamine-heavy meal) then you may benefit from taking a diamine oxidase supplement.

SUPPLEMENTS

In this massive category are an almost infinite number of vitamins and supplements, the most favoured being omega-3, zinc, selenium, vitamins B12, C and D, N-acetyl cysteine, quercetin, magnesium and coenzyme Q10. (Vitamin B3 – niacin – is also in this category but has been considered separately earlier in the chapter). Some people report fantastic results from taking just one of these (or another supplement du jour), while others report no difference.

The way I look at is that you've got a boat with a random number of holes (your possible deficiencies), and there's no way of knowing where they are. So, you are blindly patching parts of the boat in case there might be a hole there. Perhaps sometimes you get lucky and cover one up – hey presto, there's a deficiency dealt with, and you feel much better. But this is going to be a wildly different experience for everyone.

Let's move on to the next kinds of treatment, those that fall into the categories of wellness, psychological, behavioural or alternative categories.

INTERMITTENT FASTING

The theory behind intermittent fasting is that it helps the body manage inflammation, and, when the fasts are extended to more than a day, it may trigger autophagy – the process by which the body clears out damaged cells to regenerate newer, healthier cells. It may also eliminate intracellular pathogens, although the length of fast required to fully engage the process may be as long as four days.[26]

There is a vocal group of long haulers who claim fasting and inducing autophagy has really helped them, but there isn't any evidence yet showing how it works specifically in Long Covid, and there are many other reasons why fasting may make you feel better in the short term (especially if you are now intolerant to a lot of food and haven't yet eliminated them from your diet).

INTRAVENOUS NAD+ AND OZONE THERAPY

These are relatively expensive treatments that are available at some private medical facilities. Intravenous NAD+ therapy (in which NAD+ is injected into your veins) is said to help cells regenerate and aid cognitive processing. Ozone therapy usually involves mixing the patient's blood with ozone (an unstable oxygen compound) and then readministering it to the body. Used to treat infections, wounds and various diseases, it has now been suggested that it could be helpful in Long Covid. These therapies are not widely accepted by mainstream medicine as being backed by convincing science which describes exactly how they work. There is also currently no data available to support the use of either of these procedures in Long Covid – or indeed in other indications.

VAGAL NERVE STIMULATION

The vagus nerve is the main nerve of your body's parasympathetic nervous system. As long haulers, part of the dysautonomia we experience seems to result from overactivation of the sympathetic nervous system (fight-or-flight mode) and an underactivation of the parasympathetic nervous system. It has been suggested that stimulating the vagus nerve could prompt the body to move back to a parasympathetic state and thus alleviate many of the symptoms that come from spending too long in fight-or-flight mode. Yawning and massaging the ear can stimulate the vagus nerve, but you can also get electrical devices that deliver direct stimulation to the nerve. This treatment isn't as 'out there' as you might think – a team at Newcastle University have been awarded NIHR funding for their research project (PAuSing-Post-COVID Fatigue) to determine if vagal nerve stimulation is effective for treating Long Covid.

To use these devices, you connect an electrode to your ear, shoulder or neck. They then send a mild electrical signal through your skin to activate the vagus nerve. Many long haulers swear by their use as an accessory to pacing and rest generally. Personally, I have an Alpha-Stim (as discussed in chapter 7) and use it multiple times a day, whenever I stop to do ten minutes of breathwork or meditation. It's incredibly effective for me as an aid to pacing and a means to avoid post-exertional malaise. I have also found that it improves the quality of my sleep when used before bedtime.

ACUPUNCTURE

From what I hear from other long haulers, acupuncture can go either way. For some, it seems to stir up a bit too much for the body to handle, resulting in a few bad days after treatment. For others, it can be very beneficial. I was in the latter camp, and felt I made significant progress (from being in a very bad place to being somewhat functional) over two months of semi-regular treatments. Indeed, this may be something where the results are very dependent on the practitioner and approach used. If you choose to get acupuncture and happen to experience relapses frequently, it might be worth asking the practitioner to focus on one system at a time rather than pressing all the chakra points at once.

PERRIN TECHNIQUE

The Perrin technique is an osteopathic treatment that massages the soft tissues in the head, neck, back and chest, which is *claimed* to drain toxins out of the cerebrospinal fluid as well as flushing the lymphatic system. I know of a handful of people who've tried this treatment and reported positive results, although practitioners are thin on the ground and treatment can be expensive. There is currently no published evidence to support this treatment as effective, however, massage is likely to bring benefits by itself!

YOGA

When it comes to yoga, the type you choose to practise is important. Level three vinyasa, for example, is a serious workout that takes no small amount of skill and practice, and I do not recommend it for long haulers. But gentle yoga specifically intended for people with Long Covid has been reported to be very beneficial by some people.

Here the focus is on relaxation and breathwork as much as the gentle movement, and thus it could have benefits in terms of autonomic training (coaching the body to 'overreact' less to movement) and parasympathetic stimulation. If you want to know more, look up Suzy Bolt, who is a yoga teacher who has been on a Long Covid recovery journey since March 2020.

INFRARED SAUNA

Infrared saunas enable you to warm the body at a lower ambient temperature than conventional saunas, with mooted benefits including relaxation, better sleep and improved circulation. A ten-person study found that patients with ME/CFS had improved energy levels and mood.[27] It is conceivable the same might be true for people with Long Covid.

COLD WATER SWIMMING

This one isn't for the faint hearted, and requires a certain level of health before you'd even consider trying it. However, there are long haulers who have said that cold water swimming has really helped them. It can help the body manage inflammation, give the autonomic system a kick up the behind and release endorphins. I certainly found it invigorating.

GUPTA PROGRAMME AND THE LIGHTNING PROCESS

Both of these are subscription-led neuroplasticity training programmes (which attempt to reprogram the brain to take it out of a 'danger response') that aim to use neurolinguistic programming to 'hack' the brain and restore homeostasis (a state in which your biological systems remain stable while adjusting to external conditions). The idea is that these approaches break the vicious cycle whereby the body still thinks it is under attack, and thus the immune system and autonomic system can calm down, which enables healing and recovery.

To say these programmes are controversial in the community is an understatement, as there's a suggestion that simply 'thinking positively' can make you better. Having spent a bit of time with the Gupta Programme, I can state that this certainly isn't the intention, and the interventions the programme aims to make at least encourage good practice in terms of meditation and breathwork. Whatever the context, meditation and breathwork are probably good things to do in Long Covid, although clearly you don't always have to pay for them.

A small pilot RCT (published in a journal with an impact factor of 4.2) suggested that the Gupta Programme could be efficacious in women with fibromyalgia.[28] The Lightning Process was also somewhat beneficial in children with ME/CFS in a small RCT (impact factor of journal 1.3).[29] There is currently no data for either in the context of Long Covid.

CHANGE YOUR ENVIRONMENT

In the nineteenth and early twentieth centuries, people with chronic illnesses would often be sent off to convalescence retreats, often in the mountains or by the sea – an old-fashioned and romanticised idea, or one that actually has some merit? In the next chapter, I'll be talking about my experiences with this approach, and why I believe there may be something to it.

TIME

Not a treatment per se, but certainly a huge contributing factor in most people's recoveries. At the two-year mark, most of my contemporaries who first became ill in March 2020 are now significantly better than they were. Sometimes people attribute improvement to one particular treatment or action, but when you look at the group as a whole the most common factor shared by all is, of course, time.

Another important point is that time *off* may be just as important as the passing of time itself. Taking time to rest or recover, physically and mentally, can pay huge dividends. Many long haulers keep going into busy jobs under the fear of letting colleagues, patients, pupils or customers down. Sometimes having the permission to write a letter to your boss and subsequently break the boom/bust cycle of working, then crashing on evenings and weekends, can be a key factor in turning the corner for recovery.

This doesn't mean that there isn't a need for treatments that address the root cause of Long Covid – that need couldn't be more pressing. The message to take here is that if things seem really hard right now, and you're finding that no treatments are making a dent in your symptoms, the odds are that time will, in the end, be your friend.

Summary

In summary, there is still a paucity of evidence for effective treatments for Long Covid, but there are some 'green shoots' in the form of the small studies that have been published so far. As and when these findings are replicated in large-scale RCTs, we might start to find treatments trickling through into the mainstream medical community. For the time being, those of us with understanding and up-to-date GPs can still get symptomatic relief for many of the symptoms of MCAS and dysautonomia, if not magic bullets for the condition as a whole. On that note, let's address the single most important topic remaining: *recovery*.

CHAPTER 11: *What Does Recovery Look Like?*

The question all of us long haulers have been asking since the start is simple, yet profound: when will I get better? We don't have any hard and fast answers for that yet, but we are starting to see some data showing the course of Long Covid in most people. In this chapter we'll first look at the published data, then at my patient-led research, before finishing with my personal experience in trying to navigate – and overcome – the condition.

> **What does recovery look like in other post-viral conditions?**
> I feel increasingly troubled that Long Covid is not really following in the path of anything we know about other post-viral conditions: it is more common, more protracted and involves more organs and organ systems than pretty much anything we've seen before, including Long SARS (more on which below). If we for a moment put to one side the exceptional viral infections known to be associated with rather specific long-term consequences – such as EBV, chikungunya and Ebola – there is a more typical presentation of post-viral conditions. In this presentation, a person who had been through a common or garden viral infection by the influenza virus, herpes simplex virus, cold-causing coronavirus infection might experience headaches, confusion, aching muscles or joints, swollen lymph nodes and sore throat for a couple of weeks before returning to baseline health. I'm not sure that I've seen any comprehensive studies that characterise people through these periods.

One hypothesis that gets put forward is that these post-viral symptoms are caused by an ongoing inflammatory response, especially excess cytokine release, including in the central nervous system.[1] When the first cases of Long Covid were reported, explanations of this type were definitely the most prominent, and were sometimes expressed rather dismissively: 'What's the big deal? It's just recovery from a mild infection.' As we now know, that couldn't be further from the truth.

The other significant viral infections to consider in this category might all be considered special cases. We've written elsewhere in the book (chapter 4) about how most people who experience acute EBV infections normally return to their baseline health in a month or two. However, a significant minority will show quite marked fatigue and altered susceptibility to other infections for a year or more afterwards. It seems easy to rationalise such changes when considering a virus that takes up lifelong residence in a cycle of latency and reactivation, constantly interacting with and restimulating immune system B cells and T cells.

Long-term symptoms after Ebola virus infection came as more of a surprise, though. Clinical understanding of Ebola was sparse until the 2013–16 outbreaks in west Africa, and knowledge of convalescent survivors was even sparser. During that period, there were around 28,000 cases of Ebola virus infection and an estimated 11,000 deaths. Each of the outbreaks was associated with well-documented, long-term, chronic disease sequelae. These were initially termed post-Ebola syndrome and then, more commonly, post-Ebola virus syndrome. There was a really major, impressive programme to document a long-term cohort with post-Ebola virus syndrome in the PREVAIL Study in Liberia.[2]

Roughly 75% of survivors of Ebola experience chronic symptoms including headaches, back pain, arthralgia, disturbed sleep, uveitis (inflammation of the uvea in the middle of the eye, causing impaired vision), depression and muscle tenderness. Most of these symptoms, with the exception of the uveitis, decline to some extent with time, over a period of years. A possible contributor, not appreciated until years after the initial outbreaks, is that the virus can persist – for example, some men's semen tests positive for remnants of Ebola virus more than three years after initial infection. There still isn't a comprehensive understanding of what's causing the long-term illness, although induction of autoimmunity has been posited.

Considering that SARS is such a close relation of SARS-CoV-2 on a genetic level, I've been very motivated throughout the past few years to try to uncover the story of Long SARS, in the hope that understanding the trajectory of what became of survivors from the 2002–04 outbreak with persistent symptoms might offer a glimpse into the future for people with Long Covid. My initial enquiries were unrewarding. Of the SARS patients in Hong Kong, for example, colleagues I spoke with could offer no indication that there had been any long-term symptoms. I then came across a research paper following up for three years a cohort of healthcare workers in Toronto who had caught SARS that described 'persistent fatigue, diffuse myalgia, weakness, depression and non-restorative sleep'.[3]

At the time, most didn't consider the topic of sufficient clinical interest to invest in further research on it, so there was no detailed, mechanistic follow-up. A follow-up account featuring longer-term observations on this SARS cohort has been published, which looks like it offers some worrying omens for Long Covid.[4] Over a period of seven years' follow-up, some psychological symptoms continued to worsen over time, including depression, anxiety, pain and vitality. Although it wasn't a detailed study of pathogenesis, in our current situation, it makes for scary reading. The long-term retrospective on this SARS cohort concludes, 'clinically none of our 50 patients got their old life back with time and treatment. Some were never able to return to work. Some had a trial of return to work and failed. Some had a trial of return to modified work, which then failed.' In terms of crystal-ball gazing, that's not what we'd wish to see.

The data for Long Covid

In an early study by the Patient-Led Research Collaborative, which was published in *eClinicalMedicine* (part of The Lancet Group), the probability of symptoms lasting beyond thirty-five weeks was 91% among respondents. The cohort here was largely made up of 'mild' community cases from the first wave in early 2020, as opposed to those who were hospitalised.[5]

More recently, an analysis of more than 2,000 individuals who were admitted to thirty-nine NHS hospitals found that only 29% of patients recovered within a year, with many still reporting fatigue, muscle pain, insomnia and breathlessness.[6] In chapter 2 I made the point that the disease mechanism of Long Covid probably differs between people who had 'mild' acute cases and those who were hospitalised with severe cases – but complete recovery doesn't seem to be happening hugely quickly for either group.

One fascinating paper recently published in *Nature Communications* found that 85% of people who had Long Covid symptoms at two months were still sick after a year.[7] Only 7.7% of patients including in the study were hospitalised during the acute phase of their infections – a proportion that is representative of the Long Covid population in general. This particular finding is extremely important in terms of managing your expectations if you're early in the course of the condition. It essentially means that if you still have symptoms two months after infection there's only a 15% chance of you recovering in under a year.

This study also reported that of those who thought they *had* recovered in the first twelve months, 33% subsequently relapsed (although 'relapse' in this context was defined as even one symptom reappearing). The general trend over time, though, was for symptoms to ease: in the first year, of all symptoms reported, twenty-seven got less common, eighteen remained stable and only eight got more common. The symptoms that disappeared the most frequently were loss of appetite, change or loss of taste and smell and cough, headache, fever and chills. The symptoms that were most likely to become more common were neck, back, joint or ear pain, pins and needles and hair loss.

So, the *course* of Long Covid does seem to change over time, with most people experiencing remitting symptoms – even if fatigue (81%), cognitive dysfunction (60%) and headache (64%) remain extremely common after a year.

Patient-led research

I conducted surveys on how people infected in early 2020 were getting on after six, twelve, eighteen and twenty-four months.[8-11] Sample sizes ranged between 1,107 and 2,250 for each survey. On the whole, the respondents to each survey were new – around 60% had not filled in the previous survey six months earlier. Respondents were found through social media platforms, including Twitter, Facebook and Slack, and there is likely to be a demographic bias as a result. Most respondents were aged between thirty-five and fifty-four, and the populations were around 80% female.

It's difficult to compare results directly between the surveys, as we have a largely different cohort each time. Furthermore, selection bias – such that sicker people might have been more likely to respond – could be an issue. Those who have recovered are less likely to frequent the support groups where the survey was shared or to be as motivated to complete it. However, there are still some interesting takeaways.

At the six-month mark, 68% of respondents felt their symptoms had improved since the early months. The symptoms that improved the most frequently were:

1. breathlessness or respiratory issues
2. fatigue
3. headache.

At six months, the aspects of Long Covid that were the most challenging were fatigue (which 67% named as their most problematic symptom) and neurological issues, including cognitive dysfunction (41%).

At one year, 72% felt that their symptoms were either slightly or much better than they had been in the early months. The symptoms that had improved most frequently were:

1. breathlessness or respiratory issues
2. fatigue
3. tachycardia or palpitations.

Fatigue and neurological issues remained the most challenging aspects of the condition.

At eighteen months, 54% felt that their symptoms had improved in the previous six months, with only 19% feeling that they had got worse. The three symptoms most frequently reported to have improved remained the same. Fatigue and neurological symptoms still remained the most challenging elements. Notably the impact on mental health was the fifth most challenging symptom.

At two years, the proportion who said they felt about the same as they had six months earlier grew from 24% in the previous survey to 30%, and the number improving fell to 40% (although it was still greater than the 28% who felt they had got worse). One important confounding factor here is the advent of Omicron, with 43% of this total group either testing positive in the previous four months or feeling like they had experienced an infection.

Of those who had Omicron, 48% were feeling worse than their previous baseline, 33% were back to their previous baseline and only 18% were better than they had been pre-Omicron. So, it does seem like getting reinfected is bad news. Personally speaking, three months on from an Omicron infection, my fatigue and post-exertional malaise are much worse, my energy envelope smaller and my dysautonomia more severe. So, I would encourage anyone who has not yet experienced a reinfection to manage their exposure risk as much as reasonably possible.

Fatigue and neurological issues remained the two most challenging aspects of Long Covid, with the impact on relationships and family moving into the top five – unsurprising perhaps after two years of chronic illness.

What kind of picture do these results describe? A rapid improvement in the first six months, followed by more gradual improvement thereafter, with the improvements consistently slowing down over time. People *were* recovering during each of these periods, though, with 9% of the cohort at the two-year mark claiming to have recovered (it is worth noting this particular percentage is likely to be on the low side of the first wavers as a whole, given that many who recovered previously wouldn't have completed this survey).

64% of those who reported recovery felt that they had made a change that had catalysed their recovery. The most commonly cited factors were:

1. time (not a 'change' per se, but the most powerful contributing factor nonetheless)
2. pacing (see chapter 9)
3. supplements
4. diet management
5. medication.

I also asked what one piece of advice they would give to someone who has yet to turn the corner in their recovery:

1. rest
2. pace yourself

3. be patient, give it time
4. don't push yourself.

This might seem like a particularly passive list when we're all dying to do something *active* to speed up our recovery and make in happen *now*. But don't underestimate how difficult it is to do these particular 'passive' actions well when life and its demands have a habit of getting in the way. It is an excellent reminder that people who *have* recovered say that these are the things that were most important to their recovery.

Are you optimistic that effective treatments will be available, and if so when?

I am actually relatively optimistic about effective treatments. This is a discussion that harks back to our debate in chapter 10 about how to arrive at and test new treatments. I've spent my entire adult life in the world of immunology research, and I'd argue (proudly) that it has been at the vanguard of break-throughs in modern medicine, as evidenced by the many Nobel prizes awarded to immunologists. What I mean by this is that the speed of delivery of new breakthroughs to the clinic has been really impressive, in a way that often feels unlike some other branches of medicine, which, in my biased view, sometimes seem content to overlook unresolved and poorly understood disease mechanisms and rely instead on approaches more based on empirical trial and error.

At this stage, the arsenal of exciting new therapeutics, including immune modulators and antivirals, is enormous and growing fast. All of this makes me fairly optimistic that if we can pull together and harness the knowledge from the many impressive laboratory studies underway around the world to look at underlying mechanisms in Long Covid, this will lead rather swiftly into some effective treatment protocols. The big 'but' is that, from my perspective, this process will be speedier and more effective if it's grounded in the best possible evidence base and then trialled in statistically powered, well-designed RCTs, so that we can be sure what is effective.

Shuffling the deck

There's an argument that Long Covid consists of interconnected vicious cycles going on in multiple systems in the body, which create a cascade of issues that precipitate the symptoms we're all so familiar with. What are those vicious cycles? In chapters 4 and 5 we detailed the possible causes of Long Covid, including metabolic dysfunction and autoimmunity. For example, autoimmunity could start a cascade, including microclotting and consequential hypoperfusion (poor delivery of oxygen to the tissues), which means that the cells are forced to function anaerobically (i.e. without oxygen), which changes the chemical processes inside them and thus the metabolic pathways used (imagine a switch between tracks on the railway). In this way the cycle is perpetuated.

One of the other vicious cycles is without doubt autonomic dysfunction – our bodies getting stuck in the fight-or-flight sympathetic response, which then creates a cascade of problems, including an autoimmune response, which leads to even more autonomic issues.

This is without even addressing the elephant in the room – the question of whether persistent virus is playing a role. Evidence is mounting that there is a reservoir or reservoirs somewhere in the body driving these responses. If there *is* persistent virus, this begets another big question: is it just the long haulers who have it, or everyone who's had a Covid infection? If the latter is the case, that would suggest that predisposition to a certain kind of immune response is what leads to Long Covid. The fact that we've seen people recover from the condition would suggest that the body is either capable of clearing the persistent virus (if it's there) or simply learning to ignore it.

Either way, whether there is or isn't persistent virus, I would argue we need to do whatever we can to break those vicious cycles. This is unlikely to happen by adding a supplement to your regimen, doing more breathwork or pacing better – although all of those can be very useful for managing symptoms. To make a serious difference, what if we could stage an intervention on multiple fronts – body, brain and mind? Could we throw a big enough spanner in the Long Covid works to derail it and thereby let our bodies return to their natural homeostasis?

In early 2022, I decided to take a trip to the Alps, despite still struggling with numerous symptoms and being well aware of the perils of activity and exercise. I posted a film about the experience on YouTube and it ended up becoming quite controversial.[12] The purpose of the trip was to see whether a change in environment, stressors and, to some degree, diet might enable greater activity levels, some degree of autonomic reset and an improvement in energy levels and symptoms. I would have to be *extremely* careful with activity levels on the trip, and ensure that I removed all extraneous energy-sapping activities and prioritised rest.

In the end, the results were extremely positive. I think the combination of mountain air, sunshine and reconnecting with skiing – an activity that I associate fundamentally with good health – did me a world of good. I would never have been able to manage the activity levels I did in the Alps back home. So, why could I do it there?

I think a few key elements contributed, including much more time dedicated to rest, breathwork, sleep and parasympathetic stimulation. I spent between six and eight hours a day specifically doing this, compared with perhaps only one hour during my normal home routine. I was also only doing 1,500 steps a day in addition to skiing, compared with 6,000–7,000 back home. There was no work stress, no daily admin stress, no washing or shopping. No emails, no phone calls or Zoom calls. My whole pattern of thought, and indeed the pattern of illness, had been interrupted.

In cutting all this out, I freed up a huge amount of the energy envelope that I could then spend on the mountain, and, by not overdoing it, I think I managed to recondition my autonomic system to some degree (as observed by monitoring my heart rate throughout the trip – it became much, much lower than it usually was at home for any given level of activity). I made some other pertinent observations. Considering I had done literally no exercise for almost two years, I really wasn't that unfit. The autonomic heart-rate spiking on the first few days was the limiting factor, not my muscle strength or stamina. Deconditioning, in my case at least, hadn't played a significant part in my illness.

It was also a massive opportunity to reconnect with my body on a physical level, reconnect with nature, reconnect with, dare I say it, joy, and spend time doing something that made me feel exactly like the me who still existed in my head from my life pre-Covid.

I think that interrupting those thought patterns in this way helped me to get my body out of fight-or-flight mode and spend more time in the parasympathetic state where I needed to be. Perhaps the more we can show the body that doing something active does not create consequences, the less trigger happy the autonomic system will become – after all, this is the principle of the autonomic exercises recommended by Dr David Putrino at Mount Sinai Hospital in New York.

One final point is some important pacing context about the activity I undertook in the Alps. Firstly, I started off by spending just an hour on skis a day, instead of my usual six or seven. While I was on them, instead of blatting from the top of the mountain to the bottom, I skied for twenty seconds at a time, then stopped and focused on my breathing for a couple of minutes before setting off again. On every lift I excused myself from conversation and spent five or ten minutes practising coherence breathing. These measures were essential to counter the otherwise highly stimulating activity. And of course, once I finished, I then aggressively rested, meditated and slept for the rest of each day.

The trip was such a success that I decided to go back for another week to see if I could build on the progress. That trip went equally well (bar a foolish shoulder injury after trying inadvisable stunts from my youth). By the time I came home, I felt the best I had done in my entire Long Covid journey.

I believe that there are some universal lessons that might be gleaned from my experience (I know of at least ten other long haulers who have done something similar with similar results). The first part of the equation is environment. I think there's a lot to be said for switching out your daily normal environment for somewhere you can cut yourself off from the daily stresses and thought patterns that dominate your life without your even realising it. Can you get to the mountains? Or to the coast? Good weather is desirable, so if it's winter you might have to try to venture abroad. Of course, such a trip is dependent on being able to manage and *afford* the associated travel (and we know that Long Covid is particularly brutal on finances). The big point here is not to underestimate the power of fresh air and sunshine, especially in the context of a lowering of your allostatic load.

In this new environment, is there something you can do that reconnects you with the old healthy you (without, of course, overdoing it)? Unless you're an experienced skier, I wouldn't recommend you try exactly the same thing I did – it will burn too much energy. Equally, I wouldn't have been able to manage a walking holiday in the Alps, but I could stand on two planks and let gravity slide me down hills, stopping every twenty seconds or so.

Fundamentally if there is something you can do which works in the same way for you – maybe swimming, or yoga – then I believe that it could help to create a more successful intervention in breaking those vicious cycles that function on so many different levels. We need to intervene in as many ways as possible to move the dial here. How can you find that version of 'flow' and physical connection that works for you?

I do of course need to add that you need to be at the right stage of your recovery to be able to try this kind of thing. There's no point going away if the travel alone would give you a relapse for a week. At almost any other point in my Long Covid journey I would not have been able to tolerate a trip like this – I needed to be twenty months in before my energy levels would allow it. Even so, when this trip was first suggested to me I pooh-poohed it immediately. I thought that there'd be no chance I'd be able to ski, and that it would just be exhausting travel for no reason. But it turned out that the environment, pacing, discipline and resting priorities meant I could do far more than I had envisaged possible. So, if you're on the fence about whether you'd be able to manage something similar, that is something worth considering.

Summary

Is it possible that staging a multiple-level intervention like this could help to reset those vicious cycles that prevent us from recovering from Long Covid? Just maybe, yes. While this is an n=1 experiment over a short time frame, I would add that the people I know who *have* recovered did something similar – got away from everything for weeks or months and dedicated their energy to recovery, not just getting through the days. I'd also argue that calling my adventures a 'ski trip' is misleading. What almost certainly made the difference was the environment, the removal of stressors and the increased time focused on rest, breathwork and meditation. The time spent actually sliding down hills was a tiny proportion of the trip.

I do think there's something to the age-old adage of healing mountain air. The Victorians with their convalescence retreats, sitting in wheelchairs on a balcony with a blanket over their laps, might just have been onto something.

While we don't yet have concrete figures for how long it takes to recover from Long Covid, we are seeing people recover at all stages – from people bouncing back early in the condition through to the first wavers recovering at the two-year mark. Many people have described periods of being completely bedbound at some part of their journey before recovery – so if this is where you are, don't give up hope. In the next chapter we'll address the emotional rollercoaster that comes with the Long Covid experience and how managing your ride on it might give you the best possible chance of turning the corner.

CHAPTER 12: The Emotional Journey

The impact of Long Covid on just about every aspect of your life is huge, so it is not surprising that there is consequential emotional impact. What I want to talk about in this chapter is the *emotional journey* that seems to be common among people who live with Long Covid, and how the manner in which we navigate this journey can have an impact on recovery.

In chapter 7 we addressed the impact of Long Covid on mental health and introduced Elisabeth Kübler-Ross's five stages of grief: denial, anger, bargaining, depression and acceptance. Generally speaking, the first six months of your Long Covid experience will involve battling the first three stages on repeat, with the odd momentary feeling of acceptance. The next six months frequently see depression enter the mix, with anger still very prominent. It's also quite common for long haulers at this point to reach a phase where they give up on hope, having had so many false dawns of recovery. It can feel easier to give up on hope than to risk being crushed again. If this is you, know that this feeling is OK and you are absolutely not alone.

I asked the online community how they were feeling, to get a sense of how people were coping with the emotional journey they were on, and received a wide range of responses (as is to be expected). I didn't ask how long people had had symptoms for (as putting a timeframe on this journey is to some degree arbitrary – everyone's experience is so individual and will be dictated by the degree of recovery they see over time).

> *I don't have a life path at the moment. The whole thing feels so intangible, impalpable as to have no vision of a way forward. I can't plan anything. I'm lost.*
> – James Glen

> *The goal posts are constantly shifting. Sometimes uphill, sometimes downhill. With no treatment we often get worse. It's mourning another loss, constant readjustment. I accept the reality of that. It doesn't make it easier though.*
> – A Jansen

> *I can no longer live the life I had, which might be a good thing in certain respects. It is also the end of the line for those who carried emotional debt. This will need to be worked out in order to heal.*
> – Vincent

I really, really feel for James. I think every long hauler has probably at some point felt like this, and the more severe their symptoms, the longer they are likely to have felt like this for. Most long haulers describe their worst symptoms in the first year, after which some degree of remission helps them come to terms with the new reality they're in.

For me, the loss of my old life was *incredibly* painful. There was so much I valued that I could no longer do. I couldn't work in the job I felt so passionately about. I couldn't run, play football, cycle or ski. I couldn't maintain my relationships with my friends, as I didn't have the energy for phone calls, let alone socially distanced meet-ups. I couldn't even eat the food I used to love. Every minute of every day was spent feeling awful. On top of this, there was no treatment, no prognosis and no idea when or if any of us were going to get better.

The grief came out of me in waves – once I let it. Having previously experienced depression, I knew the signs for when I needed to release emotional tension. For the first year of Long Covid, almost every day I needed to sit down, put on a meditation app and cry for at least ten minutes. Letting that emotion out feels horrible as you're doing it. It's like the experience of vomiting when you're ill – really, really unpleasant. But once you've done it, there's a feeling of lightness and catharsis. Over time, bit by bit, I managed to empty my own personal reservoir of grief.

One of the things that helped me with this was, surprisingly to me, acupuncture. I saw a superb practitioner called Sam Kankanamge in London, and one of his many talents is enabling emotional release. Huge waves of emotion poured out of me in those sessions, and he recommended I work with a breathwork practitioner, Lina Salih Didi, to take it further. This experience was even more remarkable in terms of the body-convulsing emotional release it precipitated. At first in these sessions, I was hugely resistant to letting this emotion out, but working one on one with a practitioner helped me to release tension and emotion that was locked up and that I could never have accessed by myself.

Other ways of finding your way to this end result, if you feel like it would be appropriate for you, are trauma release therapy and eye movement desensitisation and reprocessing (EMDR) therapy (where memories are accessed in the presence of a therapist and side-to-side eye movements help the body re-process emotion-laden moments). Both are evidence-based methods for helping to release trauma, and I know long haulers who have done them and spoken very positively of their experiences.

Long Covid is not all in the mind, but psychology is important

In chapter 2 we introduced the theory that trauma may have a role in predisposing people to Long Covid, similar to how people with PTSD have an increased likelihood of developing autoimmune conditions (see chapter 9). This doesn't mean that we have mental scars and that the condition is a manifestation of them – heaven forbid anyone get that impression. Rather, it means that trauma has had a consequential impact on our autonomic system and we store that tension in our bodies (see the excellent book *The Body Keeps the Score* by Bessel van der Kolk[1]). Once our autonomic system is in this highly stressed state, then a complex viral infection like Covid can tip the body's autonomic system and immune function over the edge.

The final quote above, from Vincent, describes another aspect of this emotional release and grief. I have no doubt that in my acupuncture and breathwork sessions and in my personal meditations, I was releasing the emotional tension stored in the traumatic events from the previous few years and even deep emotions from child-hood. Finding that release was painful and took time (and money), but it couldn't have been more important for me personally. Anec-dotally, the people I know who turned a corner in their Long Covid recoveries also did something similar.

Everyone will have a different way of accessing that emotional tension – the combination of anger at the condition and those you deem responsible for it, the grief of losing your previous life and any previous trauma – but I would encourage anyone who doesn't feel like they've processed and released those feelings yet to do whatever is right *for them* to be able to do so (at a point when they feel like their physical health allows it). What might your personal cues be that help you release that emotion? For many of us it's like trying to find a key to a secret door. If that feels like the case for you, write a list of the times you've experienced releases of emotion in the past, and then describe the context in that situation. Is that context repeat-able? Perhaps that context is music, or psychotherapy. Perhaps it's talking to an old friend, walking the dog, or being under the stars on a clear night. If you can find your personal cues to help you get to this safe but emotionally present place, then you can unlock this door and begin to purge some of the built-up autonomic tension.

Identifying instigators of recovery can be a somewhat chicken-and-egg scenario – did I turn the corner because I released that emotional or autonomic stress, or did recovering through time and mitigating treatments enable the emotional release? My personal feeling is that it was the former, but if you are really severely unwell (bedbound, for example) then this level of health won't enable you to do the emotional work. This is where things really are brutal, and stories like James's (above) can feel like they are on repeat indefinitely.

Either way, as understandable as they may be, continuous strong feelings of anger, bitterness or frustration will be unlikely to help your symptoms. It has been well established that what we think and feel affects our body's physiology[2] – and we know that stress leads to relapses, as does perpetuating our body's fight-or-flight responses.

Once you've managed to process and release the majority of those intense emotions, it will hopefully be possible to take stock of your situation in a more objective fashion. This is the stage when you can try to 'hack' the way you think about the condition. It's my opinion that staying in a negative state of mind ('I can't do this because I'm sick, I can't do that because I'm sick') isn't helpful for our stress levels or our autonomic system. Trying to forget about the condition, even just for a few minutes a day, may take some of the pressure off. Is there something you can do without having to worry about being sick? A game you can play or a quiet activity that gives you pleasure? Often the clearing of the mind, when it happens, is a consequence of doing something else rather than actually *trying to forget*.

The goal in theory is to work up to a point when we're not thinking about being sick *at all*. But this does of course raise a huge contradiction of Long Covid: we do have to remain aware of pacing, of what we should or should not do, and how on earth are we supposed to do that when we're trying not to think about being sick? There is no perfect way of playing this game. I just know that the days I've managed to leave the condition behind me have been the ones that have reminded me the most of what it feels like to be well, and when I've put a few days like this together I've felt like I've made a massive jump in my recovery. Again, as with everything related to this god-awful condition, there is a caveat: you have to be *well enough* to be able to do this. When you're in the middle of a relapse, or your symptoms are particularly bad, good luck trying to leave them behind you. So, this is something to be aimed for on the *good days*.

What evidence is there for the impact of our thoughts and feelings on our physiology?

Professors of Immunology are definitely more comfortable counting white blood cells or sequencing genes than trying to discuss the interface between psychological wellbeing and physiology. But bear with me while I try to describe some of the more solidly evidenced findings from the research rabbit holes I've been down. A safe starting point would be to agree that there are obviously physiological markers of stress, from the effects of released cortisol (the key fight-or-flight stress hormone) to immunosuppression. I'll start with observations on the immune system, then branch out to more holistic questions of psychological wellbeing and physiology. A recent study considered the stress response in laboratory mice with raised cortisol levels, finding reduced antibody responses and impaired ability to mount a normal germinal centre response (the germinal centres are the structures within lymphoid organs that allow B and T cells to meet and orchestrate an effective antibody response).[3]

What about stressed humans? A recent study took seventy-one US Marines who had been sent on a 'Survival, Evasion, Resistance and Escape' training course. Blood tests and evaluations were done on day two of the classroom phase of training, after seven and a half days of field-based training, and after the twenty-seven-day recovery period. Levels of adrenaline, noradrenaline (another important neurotransmitter in the fight-or-flight response) and inflammatory cytokines all increased significantly between the classroom phase and the field-based phased.[4]

Many large studies that have looked at links between personality type, markers of stress or inflammation in the blood, general health and risk of death are rooted in a heuristic 1980s classification system: the five-factor model of personality. Within this scheme, people's personality traits are categorised in terms of five dimensions: neuroticism, extroversion, openness, agreeableness and conscientiousness. In one such study, which followed nearly 1,000 people up for fourteen years, higher conscientiousness was associated with decreased mortality, which seemed to be mediated by decreased levels of interleukin 6 (a cytokine that causes inflammation).[5]

In an interesting Dutch trial, 324 patients with heart disease were randomly assigned to receive usual care plus undergo a twelve-week mindfulness training programme, or just to receive usual care. Most of the outcome measures were unaffected, but there was potentially a small improvement in performance on the six-minute walk test (which, as the name suggests, measures how far patients can walk in six minutes) and significantly decreased heart rates recorded in the mindfulness group.[6]

What is the value of these findings to the debate surrounding whether particular personalities or states of stress may predispose to Long Covid, or whether entering a depressed or stressed state *due to* Long Covid may exacerbate disease pathology? There are clearly psychoneuroimmunological underpinnings to the interplay between psychological state and physiological health in the central nervous system, as evidenced by changes to the expression of cytokines and stress hormones.

We all accept the notion that periods of stress or depression can often be precursors to 'physical' illness. Having said that, data underpinning these intuitive assumptions about psychological wellbeing and wider physiological parameters of health are hard to nail down across the reported studies. There are demonstrable statistically significant relationships in studies and meta-analyses, but often the effects are rather marginal.

In some respects, as a Long Covid researcher, this lack of evidence that anyone is more intrinsically prone to Long Covid due to their psychological wellbeing or stress levels is almost reassuring, as is the corresponding insinuation that you therefore cannot somehow think yourself better by changing your outlook. It removes any risk of misallocating 'blame' to patients by psychologising what is a very real disease process, and rightly puts the pressure back onto researchers to clarify the disease process in the body to enable progress towards truly effective therapeutics. It will be evident that this is written from my specific professional background, training and preoccupation with disease mechanisms. As I write, I picture colleagues from other branches of medicine, including psychiatry and psychology, rolling their eyes and despairing at a view that may appear to lack a holistic grasp of the whole patient.

Once we've reached the stage when we don't feel like we're living in the fog of illness, we may find that we come to assess our lives and the way we live them in a different way. Long Covid is such a profound experience that we may find ourselves re-evaluating what's important to us. However, I do need to add an important trigger warning here: if you are still very sick and recovery feels like an impossibility – and I know that there are many out there feeling like this right now – you may want to skip the remaining part of this chapter, as it discusses some of the positive changes that the condition has driven for a number of people.

I found Long Covid advocacy and research so rewarding that a second career in healthcare became very appealing. I got accepted onto a course studying paramedic science, at a time when pandemic restrictions meant most of the teaching was online – and thus Long Covid-friendly. I made it through the first year of academic study, but unfortunately couldn't complete the clinical placement because consecutive fourteen-hour days bouncing around in the back of an ambulance were not compatible with my Long Covid at the time. I've deferred until I'm well enough to continue the course, but the experience also taught me an important lesson about myself and will help to direct what I do in the future, even if that isn't working in the ambulance service.

I'm not the only person who has found the experience of Long Covid transformative. Here is a selection of stories from the community:

LC [Long Covid] has paused my plans to return to school to be a surgeon, due to both brain fog and the shaking I've developed. On a brighter note, LC has made me a more compassionate person. It's also made me very aware of my energy and more selective on how I spend it and with whom.
– Laura Long

I take nothing for granted any more. Moments of joy like my smell/taste returning or being able to tolerate a coffee or a pint / cycle ride / visit family abroad again and going back to work.
– Dr Caroline Appel

I'm moving my whole family out of London. We're moving to Bristol where the air is fresher, we can walk everywhere and have easy access to the countryside and seaside. Born and bred Londoner who never ever dreamt of living anywhere other than London till I got Long Covid.
– Francesca Leon

I quit a stressful full-time job and went freelance so I could pick my own hours. A million times happier and much better work–life balance as a result.
– Lisa Ward

As hard as the recovery has been, and LC has impacted every part of my life from work to physical abilities (not being able to cycle, spent time in wheelchair etc.), I would not change the experience as I have grown so much as a person. I've found meditation and I'm much more positive.
– Rhian Thomas

Out of the suffering emerged a new life. I can't teach in a classroom setting any more but I have discovered a love of writing and have been accepted onto a course at Oxford University. Illness forced me to create a new life but nothing happens quickly and it's taken 2 years.
– Lora Shackleton

If you're reading these comments and feeling disheartened, the important takeaway is Lora's final thought: nothing happens quickly. Every day that you feel atrocious is an eternity, and the months pass like centuries. But eventually most of us do start to feel better (even if, at the time of writing, I'm still not 100%). In the meantime, don't beat yourself up for being ill. There is no *right* way to feel about it, nor is it essential to pack in your job and move to Hawaii to become a masseuse on the beach.

For some long haulers, the illness is such a profound experience that it makes them look at the cracks in the façade of their old lives and ultimately serves as a catalyst for positive change. No one would choose to have Long Covid, or even wish it on their worst enemy, but if it were possible to learn something from the experience and improve your life, even in just some small way, wouldn't that be better than nothing at all?

There is one particular response that I want to share in full. So many elements of Rhoda's experience seem familiar, not just to me but to the majority of long haulers I've spoken to:

Long Covid has been a hugely transformative experience for me in terms of how I live my life, what I deem important and what I will prioritise forever now going forward, whether I fully recover or not.

I was the type of person who rushed around constantly, juggling multiple balls at all times. I was stressed, prone to burning out, always taking on big new projects and setting myself unrealistic goals. I had a couple of health issues in the years prior, which probably should have made me realise I was on the edge of collapse, but I pushed through, kept going at the same pace and made everything a fight that I had to win.

When COVID came along I was training for an ultra-marathon, embarking on a TV career, had representation in the UK and the USA and was running my own business. I was also a mum to two young boys and having a lot of relationship stress.

To suddenly be bedbound, unable to do anything at all and thrown into a very uncertain future was a nightmare for me. I tried to fight through, spent hours every day searching for cures, took up an admin position in a big Long Covid support group and started studying to work as a vaccinator! I look back and think, what the hell was I doing?! My condition got worse of course, and I was unable to even go downstairs and make a cup of tea. I cried for weeks – kind of gave up and actually stopped for the first time in my life. Then I started to do some meditation. I put myself on a beach in Costa Rica in my mind for an hour. After that I could get up for a few minutes and felt some relief for the first time. I realised my ANS [autonomic nervous system] was completely shot, and I was stuck in fight/flight continuously. So, I started working on activating the parasympathetic as much as possible.

That's where the change happened. I'm still not well, still crashing regularly. But I've changed my entire way of life. I prioritise giving my body what it needs, instead of forcing it to do what I want it to.

I have changed my diet completely, I eat clean (mostly paleo) and do intermittent fasting. I take time to meditate or do yoga nidra every day to keep my ANS balanced. I work on my vagus nerve daily. I don't push myself or fight myself anymore. I have a newfound appreciation for the tiniest of things. There is joy to be found everywhere if you look for it. I breathe!

I have given up on all of my old dreams and I'm actually completely ok with that. I don't feel the need to be the best at anything anymore. I am genuinely happy to make the most of what I can do. Still lots of work to do, but changing how I respond to situations is key to recovery for me, as I know that stress is the biggest trigger for relapses in symptoms. I'm an entirely different person and weirdly grateful to COVID for forcing me to make these changes now.
– Rhoda Watkins

It's OK if you don't share Rhoda's gratitude to Covid – it has taken away much, much more from us than it has given in the final reckoning. But I for one do share her weird gratefulness. I have taken the opportunity to make a number of positive changes in my life, and I think that's better than the alternative.

Summary

Forcing acceptance on yourself may not be helpful if you don't find yourself at that stage naturally. Also, acceptance of the condition doesn't mean that you have to give up hope of recovery. Likewise, finding a silver lining doesn't mean you give up the desire to go back to some of the things you used to love (when your health permits). I'd actually argue that this is the healthiest form of acceptance if you can find your way there. Key to all of this, though, is processing the anger and letting it out, rather than bottling it up.

The journey of Long Covid is hard. It takes time: maybe months, maybe years. But fundamentally, there is hope. Stop striving to be the person you were *before* and instead embrace the person you want to be in the *future*.

CHAPTER 13: *What's Next?*

It may not feel like it, but in the broader context of chronic disease research, the research landscape in Long Covid is moving extremely fast at the moment. The sheer scale of the pandemic and the shadow pandemic of Long Covid in its wake have focused the collective minds of medical academia and clinical practice like never before. In this chapter we're going to take a look at upcoming or ongoing studies and clinical trials investigating both the cause and treatment options for the condition. We'll then take a punt on what the prognosis for the condition might be, balancing what we know about Long SARS against how new treatments might radically change the outlook in Long Covid.

Causality

Let's start with a major research project that one of us knows rather a lot about: the WILCO (Working out the Immunology of Long Covid) project, led by Professor Danny Altmann and Professor Rosemary Boyton at Imperial College London.

What are you hoping to discover in the WILCO project, and how might it help long haulers?

There was never a possibility that we wouldn't be desperately keen to develop a Long Covid research programme in our lab. Rosemary and I have both worked for decades on many different facets of viral immunology and autoimmune disease, and she has worked as a respiratory consultant treating chronic lung disease. From the earliest days of the Long Covid

---

support groups, we were having Zoom calls with an amazing international network of long haulers who were starting to build up momentum and a research agenda.

Our study design goes like this. When people come into the hospital, they see a research nurse who takes a small amount of blood. Because of the huge interest in the possible role of persistent virus in the gut, we sometimes also collect stool samples. Once we get the blood samples to the lab, we test them to see if we can verify or disprove some of the hypotheses for the disease process that were discussed in chapter 4 and in a piece published in the *British Medical Journal*.[1] We do in-depth analyses of various B-cell and T-cell markers to get an incredibly detailed picture of differences in immune cells and also consider immunity to SARS-CoV-2. Many people with Long Covid have been told that they may have either abnormally high or abnormally low antiviral immunity, which has fuelled a slightly unhelpful rumour mill, with people often paying huge sums of money to get tested and retested. We hope for some resolution to the conundrum out of this part of our study.

The next part of our protocol is to look for autoantibodies (antibodies that mistakenly attack our own bodies). Many other labs have started looking for autoantibodies that might help to explain Long Covid symptoms. We've gone for this on a fairly large scale, developing our own protocol to analyse autoantibodies across virtually the entire human proteome – that is, every single protein that our cells can express. It's an adaptation of a protocol we'd been developing in the lab just before the pandemic, the aim of which was to understand autoimmune effects in patients with cancer who were successfully treated with immunotherapy (drugs that remove the brakes from the immune response). The aim of our autoantibody screens is not just to build diagnostic tests for Long

Covid, but also to characterise what's happening with auto-immunity to a level where we could have some pretty good ideas about therapeutic approaches. In these studies, we'll also look at the responses of autoimmune T cells because many autoimmune diseases – e.g. MS, type 1 diabetes – are mediated less by autoantibodies than by self-reactive T cells.

We will also be sequencing RNA from white blood cells in the blood samples collected. Our hope is that by sequencing RNA across our volunteer groups, we'll shed light on what sometimes seem like complete programmatic alterations in RNA and protein expression – think of the people describing entirely new allergic profiles.

The idea is that the results of all these different analyses will come together to build tests that can really help to define and diagnose Long Covid and stratify the different presentations to clearly signpost which therapeutics should be helpful.

One of the gratifying things about the emergency of Covid research is the way that normally competitive academic re-searchers have come together. Our Long Covid research pro-gramme is strongly networked to many other studies. We'll be collaborating with the STIMULATE-ICP trial (discussed later in this chapter), with paediatric Long Covid studies, vari-ous MRI imaging studies and so many others. I hope that get-ting to the finish line on the Long Covid question will be a team event.

The WILCO study isn't the only study ongoing in the UK. The NIHR has funded a number of other projects, one of the most interesting of which is the EXPLAIN* study at the University of

---

* Clinical studies are often given names (usually acronyms) to identify them, but I have a feeling that the name is often determined first, with the compo-nent words chosen to (loosely) fit the required letters. In this particular example, EXPLAIN just appears to be a capitalised name rather than an acronym.

Oxford. The EXPLAIN study will seek to diagnose ongoing breathlessness in people with Covid who were not admitted to hospital, by using MRI scans to trace inhaled gas moving into and out of the lungs to assess disease severity and improvement over time.[2]

The US government has pledged $1.15 billion over four years to the NIH, the US equivalent of the UK's NIHR, for Long Covid research (or research into the post-acute sequelae of Covid, as they call it), although not all of this has found its way into research projects yet.[3]

One of the largest projects funded by the NIH is the RECOVER Initiative,* for a nationwide study of 40,000 people with Long Covid.[4] This four-year project intends to characterise the condition and to understand causality by taking specimens and samples from a large number of patients, as well as performing clinical and radiological examinations. It will be 2025 before we can expect to see the published results from RECOVER.

One smaller and rather more nimble team in the USA is the Polybio Research Foundation, which is investigating the possibility of viral persistence in tissue samples. It has ethics approval and the clinical and surgical teams are lined up to take the requisite biopsies. They are looking to start examining samples in late 2022. If they find viral persistence, then they will seek to understand what the virus is doing on a biological level, how it's interacting with the immune system and how it might also be affecting the local microbiome in a way that leads to symptoms. If viral persistence is discovered, then that could crack the whole puzzle open, so this is one avenue of research I'm particularly excited about.

---

* RECOVER actually is a (loose) acronym: **R**esearching **COVID** to Enhance **R**ecovery.

Which other projects are you particularly interested in following at the moment?

Normally in academia you'd be devastated if you'd moved into a research area only to realise that many of your brightest colleagues around the world were moving into precisely the same area. I can honestly say that the Long Covid urgency is so palpable that all I've seen is a great many interrelated studies with much networking, sharing of ideas and reagents, and a will to move forward fast. I sit on grant panels in various countries, and I sometimes feel I can't move for closely overlapping Long Covid studies. This can only be good news for long haulers who are impatient for speedy answers.

Horizon scanning of the big grant awards around the world reveals a number of themes: large-scale studies of cohorts and demographics (who has Long Covid and how long for), Covid immunity studies (to establish whether long haulers have immunity to SARS-CoV-2 that is unusually low, high or dysregulated), imaging studies (to look at end-organ damage and potential microclots, whether in the brain, heart or other organs), functional studies (on clotting and endotheliitis), immune studies (looking at altered immune subsets and auto-immunity) and studies to look for viral persistence (often in gut tissue or in stool samples).

Although there have already been a vast number of publications on these topics, I'd argue we're still in the early days for establishing any consensus on underlying mechanisms. I do think that some teams are doing really good things, and I'd tip them to deliver some interesting answers in the coming period. These include the PHOSP-Covid study, which involves detailed lab follow-up of patients who were hospitalised, and the immunology studies of Akiko Iwasaki's team at Yale.[5]

We need much more of this kind of heavy-duty approach if the pathology of Long Covid is to cease being poorly understood, so that it can be properly targeted by treatment or preventive measures. I'm on record previously in the book as saying that the only way to arrive at a usable protocol of what really works and what doesn't is to conduct RCTs on well-evidenced candidate therapeutics. From this point of view, I'm obviously an enormous proponent of the first, big steps in this direction in the STIMULATE-ICP trial at University College London (discussed further by Gez below).

Treatment

There are several clinical trials either in progress or being set up. All are looking to establish whether the treatments under investigation are effective in improving Long Covid symptoms, while some are hoping to resolve the condition altogether. Let's go through them in turn (there is no significance implied by the order).

STIMULATE-ICP*

This trial is led by University College London but will run at several centres. Part of the trial involves testing various medications for Long Covid, both against each other and against standard of care:

1. famotidine and loratadine (antihistamines)
2. rivaroxaban (an anti-clotting drug)
3. colchicine (an anti-inflammatory drug – see chapter 10).

Recruitment took place in April 2022, and results are expected to be published in late 2023 or 2024.[6]

AXA1125

The University of Oxford is leading a phase 2a clinical trial (phase 2 trials involve testing in a small number of patients to assess safety

---

* This acronym is too mind-boggling to spell out, and is neither meaningful nor helpful for the reader!

and gather initial data on efficacy) to see whether AXA1125 (a com-position of six amino acids and derivatives) can help to improve mitochondrial function, energy efficiency and inflammation – lead-ing to lower fatigue levels and symptom burden. The trial is randomised and double-blind (which means that neither patients nor research will know whether participants are getting AXA1125 or placebo or not).[7] Results should be available in late 2022 or early 2023.

RSLV-132

RSLV-132 is a targeted biologic drug that is designed to remove pro-inflammatory nucleic acids (i.e. circulating RNA, or potentially viral debris) from the body.[8] This double-blind, placebo-controlled study, which is being conducted by the drug's manufacturer, Resolve Therapeutics, will enrol approximately seventy patients[9] and is estimated to be completed by mid-2023.

BC007

Berlin Cures originally developed their drug BC007 to bind to and neutralise autoantibodies that are implicated in heart disease. How-ever, in 2021 they trialled BC007 in three people with Long Covid – the idea being that these autoantibodies might be present in Long Covid too. The three patients who received the trial treatment made remarkable and complete recoveries, and word spread very quickly around the Long Covid community.[10]

At the time of writing Berlin Cures are in the process of setting up a larger clinical trial. The trial is due to take place in 2023, with results becoming available in 2024.

ZOFIN

Zofin is an acellular biologic therapeutic (a treatment made using substances from living organisms, that doesn't contain cells) that has been assessed as a treatment for acute Covid infection after suc-cessful treatment of one Long Covid patient.[11, 12] The mechanism of action remains unclear to both myself and Danny. It is now being assessed as a treatment for Long Covid in a randomised, double-blind, placebo-controlled trial conducted by the manufacturers, Organicell. Fifteen patients are due to receive the treatment and fifteen will get placebo. The study started in April 2022, and is due to be completed by December 2023.[13]

IMC-2

IMC-2 is a combination of the antiviral drug valacyclovir and the anti-inflammatory drug celecoxib. Virios Therapeutics, in partnership with the Bateman Horne Center in Salt Lake City, are running a study to see whether this combination of treatments that was designed to hinder activation and replication of the human herpesvirus could have an impact on Long Covid symptoms, including fatigue, autonomic function and attention issues. Dates and timelines for this study are not available at the time of writing.

Prognosis

As mentioned previously, the closest model for Long Covid that might offer up a prognosis is survivors' experience of the SARS epidemic in 2002–04. The older sibling of SARS-CoV-2, the original SARS was a particularly nasty virus, killing 774 of the 8,096 people who caught it. What got rather less coverage at the time was the virus's long tail – with follow-up studies painting a rather familiar picture to those of us now experiencing Long Covid.

A 2010 paper followed up 123 patients two years after their initial infection.[14] The average age of patients was forty-four, and 65% were female. All patients had been hospitalised during the initial infection. After two years, 52% had persistent impairment in lung capacity, and exercise capacity and health status were lower than those of the general population. Overall, 22% had not returned to work two years after infection.

This group of patients is probably closest to a hospitalised cohort from SARS-CoV-2, as opposed to the 'mild' acute cases that lead to the majority of Long Covid cases, but there are still several similarities to what we're seeing in the community at a similar timepoint two years after infection.

One of the most recent published papers we've had during the many years since the SARS outbreak (which perhaps gives us a view into the future for Long Covid) appeared in the journal *Bone Research* in 2020. This study followed up seventy-one patients over a fifteen-year period from 2003 to 2018.[15] While the primary focus of the study was on the impact of steroid treatment received on patients' bone health, pulmonary function tests were also recorded. The researchers found that the pulmonary function of patients who did not have lung lesions in 2003 was substantially better than that of those who had significant lung abnormalities as a consequence of the original infection. Overall pulmonary function was similar fifteen years after infection to how it had been three years after infection (despite the impact of ageing). The study didn't comment on the general health level of their cohort, or any other symptoms they might have been experiencing.

A 2021 literature review in the journal *Clinical Medicine* of the long-term consequences of both MERS and SARS concluded that, while most post-SARS problems settled in time, there did seem to be ongoing symptoms, including shortness of breath, mental health issues and a reduced quality of life.[16]

Is this what the future holds for long haulers? Personally, I don't think so. The sheer scale of the problem worldwide is focusing minds and demanding attention in a way that SARS and MERS never did. If you want to be cynical, then you might have also noticed the number of *private* trials for treatments in the section above. With a potential customer base of tens of millions of people with Long Covid, there is an extremely strong incentive for pharmaceutical companies to develop treatments.[17]

So, whether we first discover effective treatments in clinical trials, or make a breakthrough on the pathology front, either way we'll be well on the way to cracking the Long Covid puzzle, and in the process hopefully we'll make a dent in the ME/CFS mystery too.

GEZ: What are your reasonably optimistic hopes for the next five years (in terms of cracking the puzzle and finding effective treatments)?

DANNY: I am a natural optimist, and a lifetime in immunology teaches you that this year's wildly optimistic research speculation can surprisingly often become next year's life-changing therapeutic. On the one hand, that optimistic temperament is quite substantially cowed in the face of the terrifyingly huge challenge posed by the uncontrolled runaway train of global Long Covid. But on the other hand, as I mentioned in chapter 10, the modern immunological toolbox offers lots of potential ways to resolve immune dysfunction once it has been characterised. As an example, I just searched to see how many different research studies are currently enrolling volunteers to trial new 'biologics' – most of these are monoclonal antibodies – in different autoimmune conditions. The answer is nearly 1,600. That's a lot of activity – a lot of research with the potential to generate great returns in the coming years.

So, all in all, I see a complex landscape over the next five years. At the moment, the number of people in the world with Long Covid is still rising, and quickly. If we conservatively estimate that 150 million people are affected globally, that's still an enormous, additional slug of healthcare provision, personnel, infrastructure and training that is required, as well as lots of people missing from work and school. Stop for a moment and consider that we've been used to thinking of rheumatoid arthritis as one of our most common chronic diseases and consideration in healthcare planning around the world. The World Health Organization has estimated that there are 14 million cases of rheumatoid arthritis globally. So, the new Long Covid caseload will necessitate substantially more doctors, nurses, radiologists and clinics. That may require some difficult discussions with policymakers about how to estimate and supply the necessary funding. For a country like the UK, this is an additional annual expenditure of billions of pounds. Then there are all the difficult negotiations about employment law and disability:

many people are leaving (or being fired from) long-held jobs because of their new disability, with all the associated effects that has on family incomes and housing. I offset the despair caused by this situation against my view that, as far as one can judge from present data, most of the physiological mechanisms and pathologies under consideration in Long Covid would be entirely reversible if we could only find those key therapeutics. For example, we've reviewed at length the likelihood that at least a proportion of long haulers may have persistent virus as a disease driver. If we can just get good at identifying those individuals, it's only a short hop from there to trials with antivirals or monoclonal antibodies, which would be likely to do the job rather well.

Summary

This chapter covers just a handful of the research projects currently underway around the world that are either looking into the mechanism of disease or possible ways to treat it. As Danny discussed in chapter 10, the research that delivers the best and most reliable results doesn't happen quickly, which means that a degree of patience is required before novel or repurposed treatments will be prescribed by your doctor. Given that none of us feel like waiting years for a magic pill, my takeaway from this is that it encourages a shift in responsibility towards ourselves. Until one of these trials starts spitting out incredible results, what changes can we make in our own lives that give us the best chance of letting our bodies find their way back to balance? How can we live more healthily – physically, mentally and emotionally? Many people have recovered from Long Covid without magic treatment, even after being ill for two years or more – and this is where I look to find the basis for my optimism going forwards.

Conclusion

DANNY: As I sit pondering my 'conclusions', we are some thirty-one months on from the description of a new viral infection. Many long haulers are well into their third year of altered health and, often, a completely altered life. All around is a rather prevalent view that the pandemic has been beaten and that we have moved on. Some people even seem to suggest that if you haven't yet managed to move on, you were perhaps getting some secondary gain from life during the pandemic. Even highly respected colleagues in medicine and medical research often reside somewhere in the 'get on and live with it' camp. This is not least because their former clinical day jobs beckon, their patients left in suspended animation and in need of some normalisation after delays in their care. Do I imagine it, or do some colleagues look askance at my ongoing obsession with Long Covid, when there are so many serious 'mainstream' medical research needs and conundrums out there? The pandemic has, in more than one Western country, taken societies that were already highly politically polarised and added Covid-libertarian versus Covid-authoritarian views into those divisions. This extends to the division between those still concerned about Covid risks and pathologies (notably Long Covid) and those for whom Covid is no longer a topic. Many of my TV or radio interviews have been followed by a certain level of social media trolling from those who are angered by what they perceive as my support for an exaggeratedly Covid-phobic viewpoint, which I presumably hold because I am a professor/bald/ugly/probably have no friends or life and so relish spending an extended lockdown in my cave!

A high degree of concern about – or even obsession with – Long Covid as a major new, global, public health issue seems more than warranted by the data. Depending on preference, the data can be narrated at the level of human interest, in personal stories of lost lives, jobs or dreams, or of schoolchildren upended from their education and social groups. Alternatively, the narrative can be conveyed in the form of big-data from national and international surveys such as those published by the Office for National Statistics in the UK, the Centers for Disease Control and Prevention in the USA and the World Health Organization. By its nature, Long Covid is hard to quantify because it offers such a moving target: new cases are coming into the equation all the time, but equally some people are leaving the caseload as the 'luckier' ones who find that, at three or six months, they can resume their old lives, virtually free of symptoms. Long Covid deniers are quick to point out that most Long Covid is 'self-reported', which seems both spurious and cruel when one considers that we still lack objective, validated and agreed tests that could make it anything other than 'self-reported'.

At the time of writing, there are perhaps 2 million Long Covid cases in the UK and perhaps 150 million cases globally. My personal view, sadly, is that these figures may be underestimates. Many people experiencing a new and chronic disability may err towards stoicism and assume that it's probably too much bother to see a doctor about it if no limbs are broken and it doesn't seem life-threatening. And of course this also supposes that everyone is lucky enough to live in a part of the world with easy access to doctors in the first place.

Even if people are immune to the human suffering that Long Covid is causing, the health economics associated with the condition – i.e. the costs detailed in healthcare-planning projections to manage the condition – should force them to sit up and take notice. The health-economic analysis of Long Covid is still in its infancy, but a long-term disease that looks set to cast a longer shadow than even rheumatoid arthritis will have massive ramifications for healthcare services, including the numbers of doctors, nurses, physiotherapists and imagers needed to confront the disease. And this is before we consider education, numbers of people in the workforce and in employment and disability legislation. The sheer scale of Long Covid suggests the potential to destroy not just lives, but also economies. The cynic in me wonders if politicians around the world are not queuing up to demonstrate their urgent responses to these horrors because they can be better kicked down the road for some future government to worry about, some other time. Long Covid is not going anywhere fast, so what's the rush?

Throughout these past years, the charge to deal with Long Covid has been led by support groups built by people with the condition, and this will certainly remain the case. The UK will soon start collecting evidence for its Covid response inquiry, and data from long haulers will be an important component in that evidence. We don't normally think about politicians taking ethical or medical decisions on our behalf, so much as making decisions on taxation policy, crime or defence, yet the decision to tolerate massive Omicron (and subvariant) spread in the UK – at one stage it affected one in every thirteen people in the UK – on the grounds that it was less often lethal than previous strains was exactly that, and it's a decision that (at this point) has resulted in an additional 619,000 people joining the Long Covid caseload, according to the ONS numbers.

My impression is that researchers have also become polarised over the past few years in their specific Long Covid obsessions. It is perhaps inevitable that expert researchers are forced to develop a rather narrow view – expertise is all about the detail. And so, we end up with fierce proponents of specific theories, whether it's persistent virus reservoirs, or endotheliitis, or hypercoagulation, or autoimmunity, or other views. As we've discussed throughout the book, Long Covid is a complex, multi-system, multi-organ disease, and we don't need to fight over a 'one-size-fits-all' answer. What we do need is to start pulling all the experts together to thrash out some consensus in ideas and a clear direction of travel for future research. Some governments have been forthcoming with initial research funding, but much of this will soon be spent, and far more will be required to get close to any kind of finish line.

Where does all this leave me and my hopes for the next few years? As I've said, I'm in some respects rather desperate that this is a massive and long-term problem with the potential to leave many lives destroyed. But, as one who has spent a lifetime studying immunology and seeing countless amazing therapeutics come online in the clinic, I remain an optimist. In that respect, if we can continue to firm-up mechanistic hypotheses and trial rational therapeutics based on those hypotheses in properly powered RCTs, I believe that we can get some really useful answers that may restore lives. This will need some real momentum. In the meantime, the interim solutions will depend on the Long Covid clinics. They are currently available in some countries but not others, with massive variations in the services on offer even within a given country. There's no point venting fury on hapless doctors who haven't single-handedly worked out a magical solution for a disease they simply don't understand without any formal guidelines or resources. Grappling with all of these challenges, some do well, others less so. Just as in other diseases, doctors urgently need to start sharing experiences with a view towards assembling and publishing some agreed international treatment guidelines for Long Covid best practices.

GEZ: The first two years of the pandemic were characterised by a mammoth effort by patients to drive recognition and make the medical establishment sit up and take notice. Long Covid is a condition that was named by patients, researched by patients and forced onto authorities' agendas by patients. While the baton has to some extent now been handed over to medical institutions, this remains a journey we are on together. As patients, we retain the power to hold those institutions – and even governments – to account. This is why it feels particularly apposite to author this book with Danny. Between us, we represent the journey that our course of knowledge around the condition has travelled, and the direction it will take in the future.

After spending months developing, researching and writing this book, it might seem like an odd thing to hope for huge sections of this book to be made redundant in one fell swoop. But that is precisely what I am hoping for in the coming months – a huge breakthrough on the research or treatment fronts that radically changes our perspective on this enigmatic and crippling condition, which does its best to defy normal testing, diagnostics and definitions. That could all come with the click of a 'publish' button by a major journal, and from the bottom of my heart I hope it happens. Right now, though, a breakthrough of that scale remains unlikely. Our cracking of the puzzle is likely to come in smaller incremental steps. As our knowledge evolves and treatments improve, I hope to update this book so that it remains the definitive resource for those who are unlucky enough to rely on it, either for themselves or for those they care for.

Indeed, such is the scale of the subject and the complexity of the condition that, while we have had a whole book to address it, somehow that still isn't quite enough space to answer every question raised by the people affected by Long Covid. If you have outstanding questions, please feel free to find me on Twitter (@gezmedinger) and ask there. I will do my best to answer.

As a patient group, our sheer, ever-increasing abundance means that long haulers remain uniquely powerful, even as the baton is passed to the institutions. Previous patient groups, such as the ME/CFS community had to blaze a trail against the psychologisation, gaslighting and harmful treatments foisted upon them by parts of the medical community. But if we can keep ourselves front of mind, driving change through tenacity and integrity as we have done so far, we can stand on those ME/CFS advocates' shoulders and make sure that the mistakes of the past thirty years are not repeated.

I am optimistic for the future, and I hope you are too.

Acknowledgements

DANNY: I'd like to thank Gez for coming up with this plan and being a great writing partner (or, sometimes, writing adversary) and, most of all, the many friends in the Long Covid support groups nationally and internationally who taught me everything I know or need to know about the disease. Also, my many high-powered Covid research collaborators, especially the amazing teams within the COVIDsortium. Most importantly, I'd like to thank Rosemary and the team at Imperial College London, who've worked more-or-less seven days a week throughout the pandemic to understand what's going on.

GEZ: If it wasn't for a rare and serendipitous trip in my DeLorean to north London's Ace Café in late 2021, this book might never have come into being. The idea had been planted in my head a couple of months earlier by the novelist (and fellow long hauler) Kate Weinberg. The previous day I had knocked my paramedic student placement on the head (it was not compatible with Long Covid, and it turns out I'm not so compatible with working in a box – either figuratively or literally), so when Kate said, 'You should write the Long Covid handbook', it was like someone had turned on the remaining lightbulbs in the corners of my brain, shining through the fog.

A pitch was written, and agents were approached. But despite interest there were no bites. I was losing heart, when a Sunday morning trip to the Ace Café for a classic car meet (and to procure a copy of *Absolute Lotus*, in which my other vehicular folly starred – an Evora S) led to catching up with two friends, Rich and Adam. I'd not seen them since before the pandemic, so over a cup of tea I reluctantly bored them senseless with tales of Long Covid woe, and the desperate need for a comprehensive resource on the topic. Adam immediately saw the value in the project and introduced me to the team at The Blair Partnership, where (unbeknownst to me) he worked. They saw the urgent need for the book too, and came on board. Under my new agent Hattie Grünewald's expert steerage, the pitch was honed, Danny persuaded to join and the first chapter written.

We then went out to publishers, and against all my expectations (but possibly not Hattie's), found ourselves in a bidding war. I don't know what the statistics are on how regularly this happens for first-time authors, but after more than a decade of pitching screenplays on both sides of the Atlantic it was an unbelievably validating and inspiring outcome.

The team at Cornerstone and Penguin really understood just how badly the book was needed and were firmly behind the way that Danny and I wanted to approach it. I want to say thank you to the whole team there, but particularly to Venetia Butterfield and Zennor Compton for having faith in us to do justice to this complex and important subject.

Researching and writing the book has been an incredibly rewarding process, as were the eye-opening Zoom calls with Danny in which we discussed the topics in question. The book wouldn't be even half of what it is without his spectacular depth of knowledge and ability to communicate the most complex of immunological interplays. I'd like to say a massive thank you to Danny for seeing the potential of the project, believing in me as a co-author, and sparing so much of his time when he is one of those leading the charge on research into Long Covid in the UK.

Writing a book while having Long Covid is a not-inconsiderable challenge, and I'd like to thank some of those in my support network who kept my dinghy afloat through the rough seas: Reena Aggarwal, whose patience, support and encouragement made everything possible, my housemate Emily Abol, who tolerated dishes in the sink and a shambles stumbling round the house, Asad Khan for his knowledge and counsel, and my family for always having my back when I needed it. My mum is no longer with us, but I felt her encouraging hand on my shoulder when the going got tough. She would be proud to have this book in her collection.

I would also like to say a huge thank you to those who have helped the book come together, either through direct contribution, advice, feedback or support. If you feel like you should be on here and I've forgotten you, I claim brain fog. Apologies.

Kate Weinberg

Joel Mishcon

Adam Reed

Sammie Mcfarland

Dr Sally Riggs

Dr Amy Proal

Dr Beate Jaeger

Dr Tania Dempsey

Professor Brendan Delaney

Dr Susannah Thompson

Dr David Putrino

Janey @ thewellnesslab.com

Sam Kankanamge

Lina Salidh Didi

Dr Tina Peers

Dr Binita Kane

Dr David Brady

Professor Todd Davenport

Darren Brown

Dr Svetlana Blitshteyn

Dr Bruce Patterson

Hannah Davis

Dr Tamsin Lewis

Sarah Graham

Dr Nina Muirhead

Professor Brian Hughes

Anke Borchers

Rachel Robins

Irma Peach

Harry Leeming

It has been a privilege and an honour to have the opportunity to represent the tens of millions of long haulers worldwide with this book, and so my final thank you is to all the other members of the 'worst club in the world'™, who have supported me on the journey so far. May you all recover faster than we can list the names of our mountain of daily supplements – and, if reading that list alone would give you post-exertional malaise, then here's to the development of a universal over-the-counter treatment that renders this book obsolete before we get to the second edition.

Look after yourselves, and till next time.

Notes

1: What Is Long Covid?

1   Hannah E Davis, Gina S Assaf, Lisa McCorkell, et al. Characterising long COVID in an international cohort: 7 months of symptoms and their impact. *eClinicalMedicine* 2021; 38: 101019.

2   Jessica S Rogers-Brown, Valentine Wanga, Catherine Okoro, et al. Outcomes among patients referred to outpatient rehabilitation clinics after COVID-19 diagnosis – United States, January 2020–March 2021. *Morbidity and Mortality Weekly Report* 2021; 70: 967–71.

3   Sandra Lopez-Leon, Talia Wegman-Ostrosky, Carol Perelman, et al. More than 50 long-term effects of COVID-19: a systematic review and meta-analysis. *Nature* 2021; 11: 16144.

4   Jon Klein, Jamie Wood, Jillian Jaycox, et al. Distinguishing features of Long COVID identified through immune profiling. *medRxiv* (preprint) 2022. Available at: https://www.medrxiv.org/content/10.1101/2022.08.09.22278592V1

5   Carlo Cervia, Yves Zurbuchen, Patrick Taeschler, et al. Immunoglobulin signature predicts risk of post-acute COVID-19 syndrome. *Nature Communications* 2022; 13: 446.

6   Yapeng Su, Dan Yuan, Daniel G Chen, et al. Multiple early factors anticipate post-acute COVID-19 sequelae. *Cell* 2022; 185: 881–95.

7   Liane S. Canas, Erika Molteni, Jie Deng, et al. Profiling post-COVID syndrome across different variants of SARS-CoV-2. *medRxiv* (preprint) 2022. Available at: https://www.medrxiv.org/content/10.1101/2022.07.28.22278159V1

8   Leonard B Weinstock, Jill B Brook, Arthur S Walters, et al. Mast cell activation symptoms are prevalent in long-COVID. *International Journal of Infectious Diseases* 2021; 112: 217–26.

9   R Miller, A R Wentzel, G A Richards. COVID-19: NAD+ deficiency may predispose the aged, obese and type 2 diabetics to mortality through its effect on SIRT1 activity. *Medical Hypotheses* 2020; 144: 110044.

10 Gez Medinger. The puzzle comes together – why dysfunctional metabolism might explain Long Covid. 13 February 2022. Available at https://www.youtube.com/watch?v=ZFPleh6z7io

11 Cameron K Ormiston, Iwona Świątkiewicz, Pam R Taub. Postural orthostatic tachycardia syndrome as a sequela of COVID-19. Available at: https://pubmed.ncbi.nlm.nih.gov/35853576/

12 Joan B Soriano, Srinivas Murthy, John C Marshall, et al. A clinical case definition of post-COVID-19 condition by a Delphi consensus. *The Lancet Infectious Diseases* 2021; 22: e102–07. Available at https://www.youtube.com/watch?v=ZFPleh6z7io

13 A. Dennis, M. Wamil, J. Alberts et al. (2021), 'Multiorgan impairment in low-risk individuals with post-COVID-19 syndrome: a prospective, community-based study', BMJ Open, 11 (3), pp. e048391. Available at: https://bmjopen.bmj.com/content/11/3/e048391

14 Q. Long, X. Tang, Q. Shi et al. (2020), 'Clinical and immunological assessment of asymptomatic SARS-CoV-2 infections', *Nature Medicine*, 26, pp. 1200–1204. Available at: https://www.nature.com/articles/s41591-020-0965-6

15 Jonathan P Rogers, Edward Chesney, Dominic Oliver, et al. Psychiatric and neuropsychiatric presentations associated with severe coronavirus infections: a systematic review and meta-analysis with comparison to the COVID-19 pandemic. Available at: https://pubmed.ncbi.nlm.nih.gov/32437679/

16 Oliver O'Sullivan. Long-term sequelae following previous coronavirus epidemics. *Clinical Medicine* 2021; 68–70.

2: *Who Gets Long Covid and Why?*

1 Carlo Cervia, Yves Zurbuchen, Patrick Taeschler, et al. Immunoglobulin signature predicts risk of post-acute COVID-19 syndrome. *Nature Communications* 2022; 13: 446.

2 Yapeng Su, Dan Yuan, Daniel G Chen, et al. Multiple early factors anticipate post-acute COVID-19 sequelae. *Cell* 2022; 185: 881–95.

3 Maxime Taquet, Quentin Dercon, Sierra Luciano, et al. Incidence, co-occurrence, and evolution of long-COVID features: a 6 month retrospective cohort study of 273,618 survivors of COVID-19. *PLoS Medicine* 2021; 18: e1003773.

4 Carole H Sudre, Benjamin Murray, Thomas Varsavsky, et al. Attributes and predictors of long COVID. *Nature Medicine* 2021; 27: 626–31.

5 Yan Xie, Benjamin Bowe, Ziyad Al-Aly. Burdens of post-acute sequelae of COVID-19 by severity of acute infection, demographics and health status. *Nature Communications* 2021; 12: 6571.

6 Cervia et al., 2022.

7 Su et al., 2022.

8 Taquet et al., 2021.

9 Sudre et al., 2021.

10 Xie et al., 2021.

11 Cervia et al., 2022.

12 Taquet et al., 2021.

13 Sudre et al., 2021.

14 Kjetil Bjornevik, Marianna Cortese, Brian C Healy. Longitudinal analysis reveals high prevalence of Epstein-Barr virus associated with multiple sclerosis. *Science* 2022; 375: 296–301.

15 Francesca Bai, Daniele Tomasoni, Camilla Falcinella, et al. Female gender is associated with long COVID syndrome: a prospective cohort study. Available at: https://pubmed.ncbi.nlm.nih.gov/34763058/

16 Taquet et al., 2021.

17 Sudre et al., 2021.

18 Gez Medinger. Can symptoms alone diagnose COVID-19? / Comprehensive symptom studies analysis. 9 July 2020. Available at: youtube.com/watch?v=24IJ2dHbYPk&ab_channel=RUN-DMC%2FGezMedinger

19 Markus Feuerer, Laura Herrero, Daniela Cipolletta, et al. Fat T_{reg} cells: a liaison between the immune and metabolic systems. *Nature Medicine* 2009; 15: 930–39.

20 Shane Kelly, Noel Pollock, George Polglass, et al. Injury and illness in elite athletics: a prospective cohort study over three seasons. *International Journal of Sports Physical Therapy* 2022; 17: 420–33.

21 Gez Medinger. Can symptoms alone diagnose COVID-19? 2020.

22 National Institute for Health and Care Excellence. Rheumatoid arthritis: how common is it? National Institute for Health and Care Excellence, 2020. Available at: https://cks.nice.org.uk/topics/rheumatoid-arthritis/background-information/prevalence-incidence/

23 Neil Pearce, Juha Pekkanen, Richard Beasley. How much asthma is really attributable to atopy? *Thorax* 1999; 54: 268–72.

24 Simon M Collin, Inger J Bakken, Irwin Nazareth, et al. Trends in the incidence of chronic fatigue syndrome and fibromyalgia in the UK, 2001–2013: a Clinical Practice Research Datalink study. *Journal of the Royal Society of Medicine* 2017; 110: 231–44.

25 Jessica A Eccles, Beth Thompson, Kristy Themelis, et al. Beyond bones: the relevance of variants of connective tissue (hypermobility) to fibromyalgia, ME/CFS and controversies surrounding diagnostic classification: an observational study. *Clinical Medicine* 2021; 21: 53–58.

26 Aoife O'Donovan, Beth E Cohen, Karen H Seal, et al. Elevated risk for autoimmune disorders in Iraq and Afghanistan veterans with posttraumatic stress disorder. *Biological Psychiatry* 2015; 77: 365–74.

27 Stephen W Porges. The polyvagal theory: new insights into adaptive reactions of the autonomic nervous system. *Cleveland Clinic Journal of Medicine* 2009; 76: 86–90.

28 Melanie Dani, Andreas Dirksen, Patricia Taraborrelli, et al. Autonomic dysfunction in 'Long COVID': rationale, physiology and management strategies. *Clinical Medicine* 2021; 21: e63–67.

29 Hayder M Al-kuraishy, Ali I Al-Gareeb, Safaa Qusti, et al. Covid-19-induced dysautonomia: a menace of sympathetic storm. *American Society for Neurochemistry* 2021; 13: 1–10.

30 Dani et al., 2021.

31 Daniel Ayoubkhani, Charlotte Bermingham, Koen B Pouwels, et al. Trajectory of Long Covid symptoms after Covid-19 vaccination: community-based cohort study. *BMJ* 2022; 377: e069676.

32 Su et al., 2022.

33 Paul Bastard, Lindsey B Rosen, Qian Zhang, et al. Autoantibodies against type I IFNs in patients with life-threatening COVID-19. *Science* 2020; 370: eabd4585.

34 Alex G Richter, Adrian M Shields, Abid Karim, et al. Establishing the prevalence of common tissue-specific autoantibodies following severe acute respiratory syndrome coronavirus 2 infection. Available at: https://pubmed.ncbi.nlm.nih.gov/34082475/

3: Can Children Get Long Covid?

1 Amanda B Payne, Zunera Gilani, Shana Godfred-Cato, et al. Incidence of multisystem inflammatory syndrome in children among US persons infected with SARS-CoV-2. *JAMA Network Open* 2021; 4; e2116420.

2 Deepthi Gurdasani, Athena Akrami, Valerie C Bradley, et al. Long COVID in children. *The Lancet Child & Adolescent Health* 2022; 6: e2.

3 Sandra Lopez-Leon, Talia Wegman-Ostrosky, Cipatli Ayuzo del Valle, et al. Long COVID in children and adolescents: a systematic review and meta-analyses. *medRxiv* (preprint) 2022. DOI:10.1101/2022.03.10.22272237.

4 Ross McGuinness. How many children have actually had COVID? *Yahoo! News*, 12 November 2021. Available at https://uk.news.yahoo.com/how-many-children-covid-coronavirus-165555811.html

5 Erika Molteni, Carole H Sudre, Liane S Canas, et al. Illness duration and symptom profile in symptomatic UK school-aged children tested for SARS-CoV-2. *The Lancet Child & Adolescent Health* 2021; 5: 708–18.

6 Dave Burke, Neil Shaw. Tillie, 11, still has a feeding tube a year after catching COVID. *WalesOnline*, 1 February 2022. Available at https://www.walesonline.co.uk/news/uk-news/tillie-11-still-feeding-tube-22941350

7 Stacey Weiner. 'Scary and confusing': When kids suffer from long COVID-19. *Association of American Medical Colleges News*, 9 December 2021. Available at https://www.aamc.org/news-insights/scary-and-confusing-when-kids-suffer-long-covid-19

8 David Olson, Lisa S Colangelo. Doctors struggle to find answers for children with Long Covid. Newsday, 4 April 2022. Available at https://www.newsday.com/news/health/coronavirus/long-covid-in-kids-cndfs9p1

9   Henry H Balfour, Oludare A Odumade, David O Schmeling, et al. Behavioral, virologic, and immunologic factors associated with acquisition and severity of primary Epstein-Barr virus infection in university students. *Journal of Infectious Diseases* 2013; 207: 80–88.

10 Gurdasani et al., 2022.

11 Gez Medinger. How to Avoid Long Covid. 17 December 2021. Available at www.youtube.com

4: *What Causes Long Covid?*

1   Amy D Proal, Michael B VanElzakker. Long COVID or post-acute sequelae of COVID-19 (PASC): an overview of biological factors that may contribute to persistent symptoms. *Frontiers in Microbiology* 2021; 12: 698169.

2   Feargal J Ryan, Christopher M Hope, Makutiro G Masavuli, et al. Long-term perturbation of the peripheral immune system months after SARS-CoV-2 infection. *BMC Medicine* 2022; 20: 26.

3   Lavanya Visvabharathy, Barbara Hanson, Zachary Orban, et al. Neuro-COVID long-haulers exhibit broad dysfunction in T cell memory generation and responses to vaccination. *medRxiv* (preprint) 2022. DOI:10.1101/2021.08.08.21261763.

4   Yapeng Su, Dan Yuan, Daniel G Chen, et al. Multiple early factors anticipate post-acute COVID-19 sequelae. *Cell* 2022; 185: 881–95.

5   Yongjian Wu, Cheng Guo, Lantian Tang, et al. Prolonged presence of SARS-CoV-2 viral RNA in faecal samples. *The Lancet Gastroenterology & Hepatology* 2021; 5: 434–35.

6   Christian Gaebler, Zijun Wang, Julio C Lorenzi, et al. Evolution of antibody immunity to SARS-CoV-2. *Nature* 2021; 591: 639–44.

7   Zoe Swank, Yasmeen Senussi, Galit Alter, et al. Persistent circulating SARS-CoV-2 spike is associated with post-acute COVID-19 sequelae. *medRxiv* (preprint) 2022. DOI:10.1101/2022.06.14.22276401.

8   Bruce K Patterson, Edgar B Francisco, Ram Yogendra, et al. Persistence of SARS CoV-2 S1 protein in CD16+ monocytes in post-acute sequelae of COVID-19 (PASC) up to 15 months post-infection. *Frontiers in Immunology* 2022; 12: 746021.

9   Kinga P Böszörményi, Marieke A Stammes, Zarah C Fagrouch, et al. The post-acute phase of SARS-CoV-2 infection in two macaque species is associated with signs of ongoing virus replication and pathology in pulmonary and extrapulmonary tissues. *Viruses* 2021; 13: 1673.

10 Guilherme Dias De Melo, Françoise Lazarine, Sylvain Levallois, et al. COVID-19-related anosmia is associated with viral persistence and inflammation in human olfactory epithelium and brain infection in hamsters. *Science Translational Medicine* 2021; 13: eabf8396.

11 Denise Goh, Jeffrey C Lim, Sonia B Fernandez, et al. Persistence of residual SARS-CoV-2 viral antigen and RNA in tissues of patients with long COVID-19. *Research Square* (preprint) 2022. DOI:10.21203/rs.3.rs-1379777/v1.

12 Daniel Chertow, Sydney Stein, Sabrina Ramelli, et al. SARS-CoV-2 infection and persistence throughout the human body and brain. *Research Square* (preprint) 2022. DOI:10.21203/rs.3.rs-1139035/v1.

13 Aravind Natarajan, Sumaya Zlitni, Erin F Brooks, et al. Gastrointestinal symptoms and fecal shedding of SARS-CoV-2 RNA suggest prolonged gastrointestinal infection. *Med* 2022. DOI:10.1016/j.medj.2022.04.001.

14 Andreas Zollner, Robert Koch, Almina Jukic, et al. Postacute COVID-19 is characterized by gut viral antigen persistence in inflammatory bowel diseases. *Gastroenterology* 2022. DOI:10.1053/j.gastro.2022.04.037.

15 Albert Martin-Cardona, Josep Lloreta Trull, Raquel Albero-González, et al. SARS-CoV-2 identified by transmission electron microscopy in lymphoproliferative and ischaemic intestinal lesions of COVID-19 patients with acute abdominal pain: two case reports. *BMC Gastroenterology* 2021; 21: 334.

16 Dalia Arostegui, Kenny Castro, Steven Schwarz Vaidy, et al. Persistent SARS-CoV-2 nucleocapsid protein presence in the intestinal epithelium of a pediatric patient 3 months after acute infection. *Journal of Pediatric Gastroenterology and Nutrition Reports* 2022; 3: e152.

17 Francisco Tejerina, Pilar Catalan, Cristina Rodriguez-Grande, et al. Post-COVID-19 syndrome. SARS-CoV-2 RNA detection in plasma, stool, and urine in patients with persistent symptoms after COVID-19. *BMC Infectious Diseases* 2022; 22: 211.

18 Jan Choutka, Viraj Jansari, Mady Hornig, et al. Unexplained post-acute infection syndromes. *Nature Medicine* 2022; 28: 911–23.

19 Dominique Grandjean, Dominique Salmon, Dorsaf Slama, et al. Screening for SARS-CoV-2 persistence in long COVID patients using sniffer dogs and scents from axillary sweats samples. *Journal of Clinical Trials* 2021; 12: 1000002.

20 Experimental Biology. Study shows dogs can accurately sniff out cancer in blood. *Science Daily*, 8 April 2019. Available at sciencedaily.com/releases/2019/04/190408114304.htm

21 Jon Klein, Jamie Wood, Jillian Jaycox, et al. Distinguishing features of Long COVID identified through immune profiling. *medRxiv* (preprint) 2022. Available at: https://www.medrxiv.org/content/10.1101/2022.08.09.22278592v1

22 Krister Kristensson, Erling Norrby. Persistence of RNA viruses in the central nervous system. *Annual Review of Microbiology* 1986; 40: 159–84.

23 Frances McGarry, John Gow, Peter O Behan. Enterovirus in the chronic fatigue syndrome. *Annals of Internal Medicine* 1994; 120: 972–73.

24 Gaetano Bulfamante, Tommaso Bocci, Monica Falleni, et al. Brainstem neuropathology in two cases of COVID-19: SARS-CoV-2 trafficking between brain and lung. *Journal of Neurology* 2021; 268: 4486–91.

25 Naama Geva-Zatorsky, Esen Sefik, Lindsay Kua, et al. Mining the human gut microbiota for immunomodulatory organisms. *Resource* 2017; 168: 928–43.

5: *The Pathology of Long Covid*

1   Inderjit Singh, Phillip Joseph, Paul M Heerdt, et al. Persistent exertional intolerance after COVID-19: insights from invasive cardiopulmonary exercise testing. *Chest* 2022; 161: 54–63.

2   Paul M Heerdt, Ben Shelley, Inderjit Singh. Impaired systemic oxygen extraction long after mild COVID-19: potential perioperative implications. *British Journal of Anaesthesia* 2022; 128: e246–49.

3   Arthur Melkumyants, Ludmila Buryachkovskaya, Nikita Lomakin. Mild COVID-19 and impaired blood cell–endothelial crosstalk: considering long-term use of antithrombotics?' *Thrombosis and Haemostasis* 2022; 122: 123–30.

4   Evangelos Oikonomou, Nektarios Souvaliotis, Stamatios Lampsas, et al. Endothelial dysfunction in acute and long standing COVID-19: A prospective cohort study. *Vascular Pharmacology*; 2022; 144: 106975.

5   Tessa J Barrett, Macintosh Cornwell, Khrystyna Myndzar, et al. Platelets amplify endotheliopathy in COVID-19. *Science Advances* 2021; 7: eabh2434.

6   Yan Xie, Evan Xu, Benjamin Bowe, et al. Long-term cardiovascular outcomes of COVID-19. *Nature Medicine* 2022; 28: 583–90.

7   Etheresia Pretorius, Mare Vlok, Chantelle Venter, et al. Persistent clotting protein pathology in Long COVID/post-acute sequelae of COVID-19 (PASC) is accompanied by increased levels of antiplasmin. *Cardiovascular Diabetology* 2021; 20: 172.

8   Peter Novak, Shibani S Mukerji, Haitham S Alabsi, et al. Multisystem involvement in post-acute sequelae of coronavirus disease 19. *Annals of Neurology* 2022; 91: 367–79.

9   Yuanyuan Qin, Jinfeng Wu, Tao Chen, et al. Long-term microstructure and cerebral blood flow changes in patients recovered from COVID-19 without neurological manifestations. *The Journal of Clinical Investigation* 2021; 131: e147329.

10 E Guedj, J Y Campion, P Dudouet, et al. 18F-FDG brain PET hypometabolism in patients with long COVID. *European Journal of Nuclear Medicine and Molecular Imaging* 2021; 48: 2823–83.

11 Chanawee Hirunpattarasilp, Gregory James, Felipe Freitas, et al. SARS-CoV-2 binding to ACE2 triggers pericyte-mediated angiotensin-evoked cerebral capillary constriction. *bioRxiv* (preprint) 2021. DOI:10.1101/2021.04.01.438122.

12 Jan Wenzel, Josephine Lampe, Helge Müller-Fielitz, et al. The SARS-CoV-2 main protease Mpro causes microvascular brain pathology by cleaving NEMO in brain endothelial cells. *Nature Neuroscience* 2021; 24: 1522–33.

13 Andrea Pozzi. COVID-19 and mitochondrial non-coding RNAs: new insights from published data. *Frontiers in Physiology* 2022; 12: 805005.

14 Daniel Missailidis, Sarah J Annesley, Claire Y Allan, et al. An isolated complex V inefficiency and dysregulated mitochondrial function in immortalized

lymphocytes from ME/CFS patients. *International Journal of Molecular Science* 2020; 21: 1074.

15 İmdat Eroğlu, Burcu Çelik Eroğlu, Gülay Sain Güven. Altered tryptophan absorption and metabolism could underlie long-term symptoms in survivors of coronavirus disease 2019 (COVID-19). *Nutrition* 2021; 90: 111308.

16 Benjamin Groth, Padmaja Venkatakrishnan, Su-Ju Lin. NAD+ metabolism, metabolic stress, and infection. *Frontiers in Molecular Biosciences* 2021; 8: 686412.

17 Gez Medinger. The puzzle comes together – why dysfunctional metabolism might explain Long Covid. 13 February 2022. Available at https://www.youtube.com/watch?v=ZFPleh6z7io

18 Britta Haenisch, Markus M Nöthen, Gerhard J Molderings. Systemic mast cell activation disease: the role of molecular genetic alterations in pathogenesis, heritability and diagnostics. *Immunology* 2012; 137: 197–205.

19 Lawrence Afrin, Mary Ackerley, Linda Bluestein, et al. Diagnosis of mast cell activation syndrome: a global 'consensus-2'. *Diagnosis* 2020; 8: 137–52.

20 Ritsuko Kohno, David S Cannom, Brian Olshansky et al. Mast cell activation disorder and postural orthostatic tachycardia syndrome: a clinical association. *Journal of the American Heart Association* 2021; 10: e021002.

21 Leonard B Weinstock, Jill B Brook, Arthur S Walters, et al. Mast cell activation symptoms are prevalent in long-COVID. *International Journal of Infectious Diseases* 2021; 112: 217–26.

22 Valeria Mondelli, Carmine Pariante. What can neuroimmunology teach us about the symptoms of long-COVID? *Oxford Open Immunology* 2021; 2: iqab004.

23 Bruce K Patterson, Jose Guevara-Coto, Ram Yogendra, et al. Immune-based prediction of COVID-19 severity and chronicity decoded using machine learning. *Frontiers in Immunology* 2021; 12: 700782.

24 Bruce K Patterson, Edgar B Francisco, Ram Yogendra, et al. Persistence of SARS CoV-2 S1 protein in CD16+ monocytes in post-acute sequelae of COVID-19 (PASC) up to 15 months post-infection. *Frontiers in Immunology* 2022; 12: 746021.

25 Anushal Chidharla, Salman B Syed, Tulika Chatterjee, et al. A case report of COVID-associated catastrophic antiphospholipid syndrome successfully treated with eculizumab. *Journal of Blood Medicine* 2021; 12: 929–33.

26 Pierre L Meroni, Maria O Borghi. Antiphospholipid antibodies and COVID-19 thrombotic vasculopathy: one swallow does not make a summer. *Annals of the Rheumatic Diseases* 2021; 80: 1105–07.

27 Xin Wang, Elena Gkrouzman, Danieli Andrade, et al. COVID-19 and antiphospholipid antibodies: a position statement and management guidance from AntiPhospholipid Syndrome Alliance for Clinical Trials and InternatiOnal Networking (APS ACTION). *Lupus* 2021; 30: 2276–85.

28 Yu Zuo, Shanea K Estes, Ramadan A Ali, et al. Prothrombotic autoantibodies in serum from patients hospitalized with COVID-19. *Science Translational Medicine* 2020; 12: eabd3876.

29 Gerd Wallukat, Bettina Hohberger, Katrin Wenzel, et al. Functional autoantibodies against G-protein coupled receptors in patients with persistent Long-COVID-19 symptoms. *Journal of Translational Autoimunity* 2021; 4: 100100.

30 Jason Laday. More than 50% of patients with COVID-19 positive for antiphospholipid antibodies. *Healio*, 8 November 2020. Available at https://www.healio.com/news/rheumatology/20201108/more-than-50-of-patients-with-covid19-positive-for-antiphospholipid-antibodies

31 Y Zuo, SK Estes, RA Ali, et al. Prothrombotic autoantibodies in serum from patients hospitalized with COVID-19. *Science Translational Medicine*, 2020. Nov 18; 12(570):eabd3876. DOI:10.1126/scitranslmed.abd3876. Epub 2020; PMID: 33139519; PMCID: PMC7724273.

32 Anthony Fernández-Castañeda, Peiwen Lu, Anna C Geraghty, et al. Mild respiratory SARS-CoV-2 infection can cause multi-lineage cellular dysregulation and myelin loss in the brain. *bioRxiv* (preprint) 2022. DOI:10.1101/2022.01.07.475453.

33 Gwenaëlle Douaud, Soojin Lee, Fidel Alfaro-Almagro, et al. SARS-CoV-2 is associated with changes in brain structure in UK Biobank. *Nature* 2022; 604: 697–707.

34 James T Grist, Guilhem J Collier, Huw Walters, et al. The investigation of pulmonary abnormalities using hyperpolarised xenon magnetic resonance imaging in patients with long-COVID. *medRxiv* (preprint) 2022. DOI:10.1101/2022.02.01.22269999.

35 Yan Xie, Evan Xu, Benjamin Bowe, et al. Long-term cardiovascular outcomes of COVID-19. *Nature Medicine* 2022; 28: 583–90.

36 Andrea Dennis, Malgorzata Wamil, Johann Alberts, et al. Multiorgan impairment in low-risk individuals with post-COVID-19 syndrome: a prospective, community-based study. *BMJ Open* 2022; 11: e048391.

6: Gender Bias and How to Tackle It

1 Joshua D Safer, Eli Coleman, Jamie Feldman, et al. Barriers to health care for transgender individuals. *Current Opinion in Endocrinology, Diabetes & Obesity* 2016; 23: 168–71.

2 American Heart Association. Why women receive less CPR from bystanders. *Science Daily*, 5 November 2018. Available at https://www.sciencedaily.com/releases/2018/11/181105105453.htm

3   C. C. Liaudat, P. Vaucher, T. De Francesco, et al. Sex/gender bias in the management of chest pain in ambulatory care. *Women's Health* 2018 14: 1745506518805641.

4   Harry Brown. Ten most common conditions seen by GPs. *British Journal of Family Medicine*, 8 July 2019. Available at https://www.bjfm.co.uk/ten-most-common-conditions-seen-by-gps

5   Laura Jefferson, Karen Bloor, Alan Maynard. Women in medicine: historical perspectives and recent trends. *British Medical Bulletin* 2015; 114: 5–15.

6   Ernest Choy, Serge Perrot, Teresa Leon, et al. A patient survey of the impact of fibromyalgia and the journey to diagnosis. *BMC Health Services Research* 2010; 10: 102.

7   Endometriosis UK. Endometriosis facts and figures. Endometriosis UK, 2022. Available at https://www.endometriosis-uk.org/endometriosis-facts-and-figures

8   PoTS UK. GP guide: PoTS on a page. PoTS, 2022. Available at https://www.potsuk.org/pots-for-medics/gp-guide/

9   M S Arruda, C A Petta, M S Abrao, et al. Time elapsed from onset of symptoms to diagnosis of endometriosis in a cohort study of Brazilian women. *Human Reproduction* 2003; 18: 756–59.

10 Tania M V Santos, Ana M Pereira, Reginaldo G C Lopes, et al. Lag time between onset of symptoms and diagnosis of endometriosis. *Einstein* 2012; 10: 39–43.

11 Ahmed M Soliman, Mahesh Fuldeore, Michael C Snabes. Factors associated with time to endometriosis diagnosis in the United States. *Journal of Women's Health* 2017; 26: 788–97.

12 Lanlan Zhang, Elizabeth A Reynolds Losin, Yoni K Ashar, et al. Gender biases in estimation of others' pain. *Journal of Pain* 2021; 22: 1048–59.

13 Maya Dusenbery. *Doing Harm: The Truth About How Bad Medicine and Lazy Science Leave Women Dismissed, Misdiagnosed, and Sick.* London: HarperOne, 2017.

14 Juul Houwen, Peter L B J Lucassen, Hugo W Stappers, et al. Medically unexplained symptoms: time to and triggers for diagnosis in primary care consultations. *British Journal of General Practice* 2020; 70: e86–94.

15 Cristina Lluch, Laura Galiana, Pablo Domenech, et al. The impact of the COVID-19 pandemic on burnout, compassion fatigue, and compassion satisfaction in healthcare personnel: a systematic review of the literature published during the first year of the pandemic. *Healthcare* 2022; 10: 364.

7: *The Impact of Long Covid on Mental Health*

1   Jessica S Rogers-Brown, Valentine Wanga, Catherine Okoro, et al. Outcomes among patients referred to outpatient rehabilitation clinics after COVID-19 diagnosis – United States, January 2020–March 2021. *Morbidity and Mortality Weekly Report* 2021; 70: 967–71.

2   L Attademo, F Bernardini. Are dopamine and serotonin involved in COVID-19 pathophysiology? *European Journal of Psychiatry* 2021; 35: 62–63.

3   Corinna Sadlier, Werner C Albrich, Ujjwal Neogi, et al. Metabolic rewiring and serotonin depletion in patients with postacute sequelae of COVID-19. *Allergy* 2022; 77: 1623–25.

4   Valeria Mondelli, Carmine Pariante. What can neuroimmunology teach us about the symptoms of long-COVID? *Oxford Open Immunology* 2021; 2: iqab004.

5   Simeon J Zürcher, Céline Banzer, Christine Adamus, et al. Post-viral mental health sequelae in infected persons associated with COVID-19 and previous epidemics and pandemics: systematic review and meta-analysis of prevalence estimates. *Journal of Infection and Public Health* 2022; 15: 599–608.

6   Simon Wessely, Anthony David, Sue Butler, et al. Management of chronic (post-viral) fatigue syndrome. *Journal of the Royal College of GPs* 1989; 39: 26–29.

7   Wessely et al., 1989.

8   P D White, K A Goldsmith, A L Johnson, et al. Comparison of adaptive pacing therapy, cognitive behaviour therapy, graded exercise therapy, and specialist medical care for chronic fatigue syndrome (PACE): a randomised trial. *The Lancet* 2011; 377: 823–36.

9   Ingrid Torjesen. Pressure grows on *Lancet* to review 'flawed' PACE trial. *British Medical Journal* 2018; 362: k3621.

10 Institute of Medicine of the National Academies. *Beyond Myalgic Encephalomyelitis/Chronic Fatigue Syndrome: Redefining an Illness*. Washington, DC: The National Academies Press, 2015.

11 Jonathan C W Edwards, Simon McGrath, Adrian Baldwin, et al. The biological challenge of myalgic encephalomyelitis/chronic fatigue syndrome: a solvable problem. *Fatigue* 2016; 4: 63–69.

12 David Tuller. Trial by error: the troubling case of the PACE chronic fatigue syndrome study. *Virology Blog*, 21 October 2015. Available at https://www.virology.ws/2015/10/21/trial-by-error-i/

13 Carolyn E Wilshire, Tom Kindlon, Robert Courtney, et al. Rethinking the treatment of chronic fatigue syndrome–a reanalysis and evaluation of findings from a recent major trial of graded exercise and CBT. *BMC Psychology* 2019; 6: 6.

14 Nadine Herr, Chirstophe Bode, Daniel Duerschmied. The effects of serotonin in immune cells. *Frontiers in Cardiovascular Medicine* 2017; 4: 48.

15 Gez Medinger. The Why When and How of Pacing. 13 July 2021. Available at https://www.youtube.com/watch?v=gUPvNwvkOlA

16 Matthew Walker. *Why We Sleep: The New Science of Sleep and Dreams*. London: Simon & Schuster, 2017.

17 Heidi L Heard, Marsha M Linehan. Dialectical behavior therapy: an integrative approach to the treatment of borderline personality disorder. *Journal of Psychotherapy Integration* 1994; 4: 55–82.

8: *How to Help Others Help You*

1   Martine Nurek, Clare Rayner, Anette Freyer, et al. Recommendations for the recognition, diagnosis, and management of long COVID: a Delphi study. *British Journal of General Practice* 2021; 71: e815–20.

2   Office for National Statistics. Prevalence of ongoing symptoms following coronavirus (COVID-19) infection in the UK: 1 June 2022. Office for National Statistics, 1 June 2022. Available at https://www.ons.gov.uk/peoplepopulationandcommunity/healthandsocialcare/conditionsanddiseases/bulletins/prevalenceofongoingsymptomsfollowingcoronaviruscovid19infectionintheuk/1june2022

3   Infographic: Bodily Systems Affected by Long COVID. Available at: https://www.the-scientist.com/infographics/infographic-bodily-systems-affected-by-long-covid-69083

9: *Tips for Managing Symptoms*

1   Emilia Sforza, David Hupin, Frédéric Roche. Mononucleosis: a possible cause of idiopathic hypersomnia. *Frontiers in Neurology* 2018; 9: 922.

2   Kellen Mulhern. 1261 the long term exhaustion of a viral infection. *Sleep* 2021; 43: A480.

3   Dan Hurley. Sleep neurologists call it 'COVID-somnia'–increased sleep disturbances linked to the pandemic. *NeurologyToday*, 9 July 2020. Available at https://journals.lww.com/neurotodayonline/fulltext/2020/07090/sleep_neurologists_call_it.1.aspx

4   Gerwyn Morris, George Anderson, Michael Maes. Hypothalamic-pituitary-adrenal hypofunction in myalgic encephalomyelitis (ME)/chronic fatigue syndrome (CFS) as a consequence of activated immune-inflammatory and oxidative and nitrosative pathways. *Molecular Neurobiology* 2016; 54: 6806–19.

5   Matthew Walker. *Why We Sleep: The New Science of Sleep and Dreams*. London: Simon & Schuster, 2017.

6   Christine Miserandino. The spoon theory. *ButYouDon'tLookSick*, 2003. Available at https://butyoudontlooksick.com/articles/written-by-christine/the-spoon-theory/

7   Paul Garner. Covid-19 at 14 weeks–phantom speed cameras, unknown limits, and harsh penalties. *BMJ Opinion*, 23 June 2020. Available at https://

blogs.bmj.com/bmj/2020/06/23/paul-garner-covid-19-at-14-weeks-phantom-speed-cameras-unknown-limits-and-harsh-penalties/

8 Elden Berla Thangam, Ebenezer Angel Jemima, Himadri Singh, et al. The role of histamine and histamine receptors in mast cell-mediated allergy and inflammation: the hunt for new therapeutic targets. *Frontiers in Immunology* 2018; 9: 1873.

9 Laura Maintz, Natalija Novak. Histamine and histamine intolerance. *The American Journal of Clinical Nutrition* 2007; 85: 1185–96.

10 Gez Medinger. First effective treatment for Long Covid | Stunning data from huge new study. 22 December 2020. Available at https://www.youtube.com/watch?v=9-3V3honcIA

11 Marisa E Hilliard, Joyce P Yi-Frazier, Danielle Hessler, et al. Stress and A1c among people with diabetes across the lifespan. *Current Diabetes Reports* 2016; 16: 67.

12 Joel E Dimsdale. Psychological stress and cardiovascular disease. *Journal of the American College of Cardiology* 2008; 51: 1237–46.

13 Habib Yaribeygi, Yunes Panehi, Hedayay Sahraei, et al. The impact of stress on body function: a review. *EXCLI Journal* 2017; 16: 1057–72.

14 Ronald Glaser, Janice Kiecolt-Glaser. Stress-induced immune dysfunction: implications for health. *Nature Reviews Immunology* 2005; 5: 243–51.

15 Huan Song, Fang Fang, Gunnar Tomasson, et al. Association of stress-related disorders with subsequent autoimmune disease. *Journal of the American Medical Association* 2018; 319: 2388–400.

16 Aoife O'Donovan, Beth E Cohen, Karen H Seal, et al. Elevated risk for auto-immune disorders in Iraq and Afghanistan veterans with posttraumatic stress disorder. *Biological Psychiatry* 2014; 77: 365–74.

17 Jamie Wood, Laura Tabacof, Jenna Tosto-Mancuso, et al. Levels of end-tidal carbon dioxide are low despite normal respiratory rate in individuals with long COVID. *Journal of Breath Research* 2021; 16: 017101.

18 Erin Hopkins, Terrence Sanvictores, Sandeep Sharma. Physiology, acid base balance. *StatPearls*, 14 September 2021. Available at https://www.ncbi.nlm.nih.gov/books/NBK507807/

10: *What about Treatment?*

1 Robert Thomas, Madeline Williams, Jeffrey Aldous, et al. A randomised, double-blind, placebo-controlled trial evaluating concentrated phytochemical-rich nutritional capsule in addition to a probiotic capsule on clinical outcomes among individuals with COVID-19–the UK Phyto-V Study. *COVID* 2022; 2: 433–49.

2 Asa Hakansson, Goran Molin. Gut microbiota and inflammation. *Nutrients* 2011; 3: 637–82.

3   R K Rao, G Samak. Protection and restitution of gut barrier by probiotics: nutritional and clinical implications. *Current Nutrition and Food Science* 2013; 9: 99–107.

4   Sammy Heung. Hong Kong team develops test for Long Covid so recovered patients can tell if trouble lies ahead. *South China Morning Post*, 11 April 2022. Available at https://www.scmp.com/news/hong-kong/health-environment/ article/3173759/hong-kong-team-develops-test-long-covid-so

5   Paul Glynne, Natasha Tahmasedi, Vanya Grant, et al. Long COVID following mild SARS-CoV-2 infection: characteristic T cell alterations and response to antihistamines. *Journal of Investigative Medicine* 2022; 70: 61–67.

6   Gez Medinger. Here's how you treat Long Covid | Lessons from MCAS – Dr Tina Peers. 24 November 2020. Available at https://www.youtube.com/ watch?v=sICD0Kn6pR4

7   S Charfeddine, H I Jadjamor, S Torjmen, et al. Sulodexide in the treatment of patients with long COVID 19 symptoms and endothelial dysfunction: the results of TUN-EndCOV study. *Archives of Cardiovascular Diseases Supplements* 2022; 14: 127.

8   Tim Robbins, Michael Gonevski, Cain Clark, et al. Hyperbaric oxygen therapy for the treatment of long COVID: early evaluation of a highly promising intervention. *Clinical Medicine* 2021; 21: e629–32.

9   Luke D Liu, Deborah L Duricka. Stellate ganglion block reduces symptoms of Long COVID: a case series. *Journal of Neuroimmunology* 2022; 362: 577784.

10 Etheresia Pretorius, Chantelle Venter, Gert J Laubscher et al. Combined triple treatment of fibrin amyloid microclots and platelet pathology in individuals with long COVID/ post-acute sequelae of COVID-19 (PASC) can resolve their persistent symptoms. *Research Square* (preprint) 2022. DOI:10.21203/rs.3.rs-1205453/v2.

11 Bruce Patterson, Ram Yogendra, José Guevara-Coto, et al. Targeting the monocytic-endothelial-platelet axis with maraviroc and pravastatin as a therapeutic option to treat Long COVID/ post-acute sequelae of COVID (PASC). *Research Square* (preprint) 2022. DOI:10.21203/rs.3.rs-1344323/v1.

12 Bruce K Patterson, Jose Guevara-Coto, Ram Yogendra, et al. Immune-based prediction of COVID-19 severity and chronicity decoded using machine learning. *Frontiers in Immunology* 2021; 12: 700782.

13 Gustavo Aguirre-Chang, Eduardo C Saavedra, Maneul Yui, et al. Post-acute or prolonged COVID-19: ivermectin treatment for patients with persistent symptoms. *Zenodo* (preprint) 2020. DOI:10.5281/zenodo.4058612.

14 Gez Medinger. First effective treatment for Long Covid | Stunning data from huge new study. 22 December 2020. Available at https://www.youtube. com/watch?v=9-3V3honcIA

15 National Institute for Health and Care Excellence. Nicotinic acid. *British National Formulary*, 13 June 2022. Available at https://bnf.nice.org.uk/drug/nicotinic-acid.html

16 Plinio Cirillo, Vittirio Taglialatela, Grazia Pellegrino, et al. Effects of colchicine on platelet aggregation in patients on dual antiplatelet therapy with aspirin and clopidogrel. *Journal of Thrombosis and Thrombolysis* 2020; 50: 468–72.

17 RCSI. Blood clotting may be the root cause of Long COVID syndrome, research shows. *Science Daily*, 16 August 2021. Available at https://www.sciencedaily.com/releases/2021/08/210816125717.htm

18 Elisabeth Mahase. Covid-19: Pfizer's paxlovid is 89% effective in patients at risk of serious illness, company reports. *British Medical Journal* 2021; 375: n2713.

19 A Zollner, R Koch, A Jukic, et al. Postacute COVID-19 is Characterized by Gut Viral Antigen Persistence in Inflammatory Bowel Diseases. *Gastroenterology*, August 2022. Aug; 163(2):495-506.e8. DOI:10.1053/j.gastro.2022.04.037. Epub 1 May 2022. PMID: 35508284; PMCID: PMC9057012.

20 Jarred Younger, Luke Parkitny, David McLain. The use of low-dose naltrexone (LDN) as a novel anti-inflammatory treatment for chronic pain. *Clinical Rheumatology* 2014; 33: 451–59.

21 Karin Due Bruun, Kirstine Amris, Henrik B Vagter, et al. Low-dose naltrexone for the treatment of fibromyalgia: protocol for a double-blind, randomized, placebo-controlled trial. *Trials* 2021; 22: 804.

22 Monica J Bolton, Bryan P Chapman, Harm Van Marwijk. Low-dose naltrexone as a treatment for chronic fatigue syndrome. *BMJ Case Reports* 2020; 13: e232502.

23 AgelessRx. Pilot study into LDN and NAD+ for treatment of patients with post-COVID-19 syndrome. *ClinicalTrials.gov*, 27 October 2020. Available at https://clinicaltrials.gov/ct2/show/NCT04604704

24 Angus Mackay. A paradigm for post-Covid-19 fatigue syndrome analogous to ME/CFS. *Frontiers in Neurology* 2021; 12: 701419.

25 Elizabeth Iveson. Feasibility of cannabidiol for the treatment of Long COVID. *ClinicalTrials.gov*, 13 June 2022. Available at https://clinicaltrials.gov/ct2/show/NCT04997395

26 C. P. Davis. How Long Do You Need to Fast for Autophagy? MedicineNet, 22 March 2021. Available at https://www.medicinenet.com/how_long_do_you_need_to_fast_for_autophagy/article.htm

27 Yuji Soejima, Takao Munemoto, Akinori Masuda, et al. Effects of Waon therapy on chronic fatigue syndrome: a pilot study. *Internal Medicine* 2015; 53: 333–38.

28 Juan P Sanabria-Mazo, Jesus Montero-Marin, Albert Feliu-Soler, et al. Mindfulness-based program plus amygdala and insula retraining (MAIR) for the treatment of women with fibromyalgia: a pilot randomized controlled trial. *Journal of Clinical Medicine* 2020; 9: 3246.

29 Esther M Crawley, Daisy M Gaunt, Kirsty Garfield, et al. Clinical and cost-effectiveness of the Lightning Process in addition to specialist medical care for paediatric chronic fatigue syndrome: randomised controlled trial. *Archives of Disease in Childhood* 2018; 103: 155–64.

11: *What Does Recovery Look Like?*

1 Masanori Yamato, Yosky Kataoka. Fatigue sensation following peripheral viral infection is triggered by neuroinflammation: who will answer these questions? *Neural Regeneration Research* 2015; 10: 203–04.

2 PREVAIL III Study Group. A longitudinal study of Ebola sequelae in Liberia. *New England Journal of Medicine* 2019; 380: 924–34.

3 Harvey Moldofsky, John Patcai. Chronic widespread musculoskeletal pain, fatigue, depression and disordered sleep in chronic post-SARS syndrome; a case-controlled study. *BMC Neurology* 2011; 11: 37.

4 John Patcai. Is 'Long Covid' similar to 'Long SARS'? *Oxford Open Immunology* 2022; 3: iqac002.

5 Hannah E Davis, Gina S Assaf, Lisa McCorkell, et al. Characterising Long COVID in an international cohort: 7 months of symptoms and their impact. *eClinicalMedicine* 2021; 38: 101019.

6 Robin McKie. Only 29% of UK COVID hospital patients recover within a year. *The Guardian*, 24 April 2022. Available at https://www.theguardian.com/world/2022/apr/24/only-29-of-uk-covid-hospital-patients-recover-within-a-year

7 Viet-Thi Tran, Raphaël Porcher, Isabelle Pane, et al. Course of post COVID-19 disease symptoms over time in the ComPaRe long COVID prospective e-cohort. *Nature Communications* 2022; 13: 1812.

8 Gez Medinger. Can symptoms alone diagnose COVID-19? / Comprehensive symptom studies analysis. 9 July 2020. Available at https://www.youtube.com/watch?v=24IJ2dHbYPk

9 Gez Medinger. Long Covid: one year in | How many have recovered? Comprehensive new study analysed. 2 April 2021. Available at https://www.youtube.com/watch?v=Ox1c10VsQoM

10 Gez Medinger. Long Covid at 18 months | How many have recovered – and what's their secret? 25 October 2021. Available at https://www.youtube.com/watch?v=cKreDsa_GqM

11 Gez Medinger. Long Covid at two years: how many have recovered? 13 May 2022. Available at https://www.youtube.com/watch?v=aJokJnBLOMw

12 Gez Medinger. The great experiment: can activity play a role in Long Covid recovery? 19 January 2022. Available at https://www.youtube.com/watch?v=UCJhYAQ6aGk

12: *The Emotional Journey*

1   Bessel van der Kolk. *The Body Keeps the Score: Mind, Brain and Body in the Transformation of Trauma*. London: Penguin Books, 2015.

2   Thibault Renoir, Kyoko Hasebe, Laura Gray. Mind and body: how the health of the body impacts on neuropsychiatry. *Frontiers in Pharmacology* 2013; 4: 158.

3   Weiguo Sun, Linxia Zhang, Lejian Lin, et al. Chronic psychological stress impairs germinal center response by repressing miR-155. *Brain, Behaviour & Immunity* 2019; 76: 48–60.

4   Alyssa N Varanoske, Holly L McClung, John J Sepowitz, et al. Stress and the gut-brain axis: cognitive performance, mood state, and biomarkers of blood-brain barrier and intestinal permeability following severe physical and psychological stress. *Brain, Behaviour & Immunity* 2022; 101: 383–93.

5   Páraic S O'Súilleabháin, Nicholas A Turiano, Denis Gerstorf, et al. Personality pathways to mortality: Interleukin-6 links conscientiousness to mortality risk. *Brain, Behaviour & Immunity* 2021; 93: 238–44.

6   John O Younge, Machteld F Wery, Rinske A Gotink, et al. Web-based mindfulness intervention in heart disease: a randomized controlled trial. *PLoS One* 2015; 10: e0143843.

13: *What's Next?*

1   Danny M Altmann, Rosemary J Boyton. Decoding the unknowns in Long Covid. *British Medical Journal* 2021; 372: n132.

2   University of Oxford. New research studies to help diagnose and treat Long Covid funded by NIHR. University of Oxford, 19 July 2021. Available at https://www.ox.ac.uk/news/2021-07-19-new-research-studies-help-diagnose-and-treat-long-covid-funded-nihr

3   National Institutes of Health. NIH launches new initiative to study 'Long Covid'. National Institutes of Health, 23 February 2021. Available at https://www.nih.gov/about-nih/who-we-are/nih-director/statements/nih-launches-new-initiative-study-long-covid

4   Lisa Winder. NIH grants $470 million for study of Long Covid. *The Scientist*, 16 September 2021. Available at https://www.the-scientist.com/news-opinion/nih-grants-470-million-for-study-of-long-covid-69192

5   Eric Song, Christopher M Bartley, Ryan D Chow, et al. Divergent and self-reactive immune responses in the CNS of COVID-19 patients with neurological symptoms. *Cell Reports Medicine* 2021; 2: 100288.

6 STIMULATE-ICP. About the STIMULATE-ICP study. STIMULATE-ICP, 2022. Available at https://www.stimulate-icp.org/about

7 Axcella. AXA1125 now in phase 2a and 2b development. Axcella, 13 June 2022. Available at https://axcellatx.com/pipeline/axa1125/

8 Kezia Parkins. Resolve Therapeutics to start phase II trial of RSLV-132 for Long Covid. *Clinical Trials Arena*, 24 June 2021. Available at https://www.clinicaltrialsarena.com/news/resolve-therapeutics-to-start-phase-ii-trial-of-rslv-132-for-long-covid/

9 Resolve Therapeutics. Phase 2 study of RSLV-132 in subjects with Long COVID. *ClinicalTrials.gov*, 25 June 2021. Available at https://clinicaltrials.gov/ct2/show/NCT04944121

10 Cort Johnson. Berlin Cures …? Could BC 007 help with Long COVID and ME/CFS? *Health Rising*, 30 December 2021. Available at https://www.healthrising.org/blog/2021/12/30/bc-007-berlin-cures-long-covid-chronic-fatigue-syndrome/

11 DrugBank Online. Zofin. DrugBank Online, 13 June 2022. Available at https://go.drugbank.com/drugs/DB16519

12 Maria Ines Mitrani, Michael A Bellio, Allen Meglin, et al. Treatment of a COVID-19 long hauler with an amniotic fluid-derived extracellular vesicle biologic. *Respir Med Case Rep* 2021; 34: 101502.

13 Organicell Regenerative Medicine. Zofin to treat COVID-19 long haulers. *ClinicalTrials.gov*, 14 April 2022. Available at https://clinicaltrials.gov/ct2/show/NCT05228899

14 Jenny C Ngai, Fanny W Ko, Susanna S Ng, et al. The long-term impact of severe acute respiratory syndrome on pulmonary function, exercise capacity and health status. *Respirology* 2010; 15: 543–50.

15 Peixun Zhang, Jia Li, Huixin Liu, et al. Long-term bone and lung consequences associated with hospital-acquired severe acute respiratory syndrome: a 15-year follow-up from a prospective cohort study. *Bone Research* 2020; 8: 8.

16 Oliver O'Sullivan. Long-term sequelae following previous coronavirus epidemics. *Clinical Medicine* 2021; 21: e68–70.

17 Carolyn Crist. More than 100 million people worldwide have or had Long COVID: study. *WebMD*, 18 November 2021. Available at https://www.webmd.com/lung/news/20211118/millions-worldwide-long-covid-study

Resources

General

- Gez's YouTube channel with over eighty videos on Long Covid: www.youtube.com/rundmc1
- The Long Covid Kids website: www.longcovidkids.org

Chapter 3

Q&A WITH SAMMIE MCFARLAND, FOUNDER, LONG COVID KIDS

GEZ: What are the options for kids who can't attend school?

SAMMIE: I've just set up a Long Covid Kids school pilot, which has teachers trained to understand, identify and cater for children with Long Covid. If you have cognitive issues, you can't just be at home and study. You have to study in an entirely different way. You need screen breaks, you need shorter lessons, and you need to know the content in advance so that you can consider it. You need to know where to go to ask questions and not feel like you're an 'idiot' for asking them, which is how the kids tell us they feel. This is happening in schools now.

Imagine how hard it is for a child to get to school late (due to Long Covid), knowing that everyone's going to judge them or laugh at them. Just walking in as a teenager anyway is hard enough if you're late to a class, and then the teacher says, 'Oh, nice of you to drop in' or 'Oh, going to pop in today, are you? Just a flying visit, is it?' This is the mentality that our kids have to address and work with. So what we're doing is providing a safe environment that allows them to work with teachers who get it.

They don't have the additional stress of ridicule. If they're achieving well one day, and then struggling the next, it's OK, because the teacher will understand, and they're not going to be made to feel bad for that. In fact, they're going to be celebrated for pitching up and trying, which in itself is an achievement. And then there's an online programme option, so that if they start the lesson well, but then get jaded during the lesson, they can actually then watch or listen back to the lesson at any time they want, and review the lesson as many times as they need to help them get the information they need. Or they could just fast-forward to a bit that they were not sure about. So, it helps to build confidence in their self-esteem, and in their ability to learn. It reduces the impact on their mental health. And hopefully, as, when and if they recover, they will have that foundation there to then build on and to continue their education.

At the moment this school is a pilot scheme, but by the time this book is published I'm hoping that we'll have made some serious inroads with the government, and there's hopes of rolling this out more widely.

GEZ: How can we help kids with Long Covid remain socially active?

SAMMIE: We've created a platform called ChatBox, which is a secure online chatroom that connects children with other children living with Long Covid. It has separate channels for different age groups so that it's age-appropriate. At the moment, we're going for ages eight to eleven, twelve to fourteen, and then fifteen plus. Then we have a parents' and carers' channel, and we're hoping to develop a teachers' one, so as teachers start identifying more of this in the classroom, they can connect with other teachers that way as well.

GEZ: What resources are there for parents?

SAMMIE: We've launched a support guide on our website. It contains everything families need to know and will continue to evolve as we learn more. It includes lived experience, signposting and information on how you get referred, who is out there to support you and which organisations can help. It helps answer questions such as, 'What are you entitled to?', 'What educational provision is there?' and 'How do you access that?' There's a section about the language children use to describe Long Covid. If you have a little kid, they often say they're 'floppy', but what they mean is that they have post-exertional malaise.

We've got resources for wellbeing, we've provided information on how to help children engage the parasympathetic nervous response, we've got a section with appropriate information for children to learn more, and a reminder that caregivers need to care for themselves too. All of that is in there, plus information for teachers and healthcare professionals. It's basically saying, 'Look, this is the reality. This is what we know, this is what we don't know, this is the anecdotal evidence that we're concerned about and these are the things that we've learnt over the last two years about what works or doesn't work.'

GEZ: What can you do to help a child with Long Covid?

SAMMIE: You can get informed early, using our support guide.

- Cautious Tortoise: an easy-to-follow flow chart that helps parents and guardians navigate the early steps of their child's recovery. Available at: https://www.longcovidkids. org/post/long-covid-recovery-for-children-cautious-tortoise

Chapter 8

- Resource for GPs not familiar with Long Covid in the *British Journal of General Practice*: Martine Nurek, Clare Rayner, Anette Freyer, et al. Recommendations for the recognition, diagnosis, and management of Long Covid: a Delphi study. *British Journal of General Practice* 2021; 71: e815–20.
- Template for headache diary, from the National Headache Foundation, which can be adjusted for use with any symptoms.

A headache diary consists of tracking the following information:

DATE	TIME (start/finish)	INTENSITY rate 1–10 (most severe being 10)	PRECEDING SYMPTOMS	TRIGGERS	MEDICATION (and dosage)	RELIEF (complete/moderate/none)

DIRECT ADVICE FOR GPS, FROM PROFESSOR BRENDAN DELANEY
AND DR SUSANNAH THOMPSON

- Listen carefully to your patient. I know we all think we do
  this, but remember this is a complicated multi-system
  disease, and you may need to offer double or even triple
  appointments to those who are more unwell.
- Screen all your Long Covid patients for post-exertional
  malaise. If they're having good and bad days with post-
  exertional malaise, then offer advice on rest and pacing, as
  early advice like this can reduce the severity of the illness.
  There is emerging evidence that aerobic exercise can make
  post-exertional malaise worse, but toning exercise without
  raising the heart rate can improve and maintain muscle
  function without triggering it. Gentle yoga, tai chi and
  Pilates are preferable to aerobic exercise in these patients.
- Education about dysautonomia and PoTS is useful as they're
  very common in Long Covid and easily missed. Be aware
  that some patients who present with palpitations, lighthead-
  edness and breathlessness that have no other clear pathology
  may well be dysautonomic, and should be treated as such.
- Be very careful not to put your patients into familiar
  diagnostic boxes such as anxiety or asthma (e.g. when
  presenting with shortness of breath). Look at the bigger
  picture.
- Know which of your local cardiology, respiratory and
  neurology specialists are interested in Long Covid.
- Consider organ damage and whether your patient needs
  referring to a different specialty. Think carefully
  through each symptom and don't just attribute them to
  Long Covid without thinking further about whether
  they need referring to cardiology for their palpitations or
  a respiratory specialist for shortness of breath.
- Don't label your patients as having a functional illness just
  because you don't understand it. Patients experienced this

early in the pandemic and it delayed treatment and was highly distressing in the process.

- If you suspect PoTS, do a NASA lean test (see the PoTS UK website) and start treatment ladder (self-help, fluids, salt, compression, consider beta blockers, ivabradine, fludrocortisone or midodrine). If unfamiliar with these, try an Advice and Guidance request to a PoTS specialist.
- Screen for mast cell overactivity and use Darier's sign. Consider a trial of off-label double dose of H1 and H2 receptor blockade – at least a month trial. Watch out for weight gain on high-dose H1 blockers – monitor patient.
- Be aware of local Long Covid services, what they do and how long the waiting list is. Some provide good medical supervision, in which case check referral criteria and highlight any specific medical concerns. Others are therapist-only 'rehab services' – don't expect anything more than this, and avoid referral to any that do not adequately screen for post-exertional malaise, use any form of graded exercise therapy or offer CBT as anything other than a supportive therapy.
- Be aware of good self-help resources for patients. The one produced by Dr Harsha Master (available from Hertfordshire Community NHS Trust) is especially good on pacing and on breathing routines for dysfunctional breathing.
- Code all patients appropriately with 'post-Covid condition' on their problem list – this aids research and audit as well as providing a proper ongoing diagnosis. Add any new conditions such as myocarditis or PoTS too.
- With patients unable to work, support with 'fit notes', be prepared to signpost and support occupational health with prolonged and flexible 'return to work' strategies.

Chapter 9

BREATHWORK
- Some useful tools to get you started are the Flourish app by breathwork practitioner Richie Bostock, which is excellent (and free, for basic access), as are the Stasis breathing tools as recommended by Dr David Putrino's clinic at Mt Sinai in New York.
- Other good apps for breathwork and meditation are Headspace, Calm and Insight Timer.

DYSAUTONOMIA
- Insight into autonomic conditioning with Dr David Putrino: Gez Medinger. The Mt Sinai Recovery Plan for Long Covid | With David Putrino. YouTube, 2021. Available at https://www.youTube.com/watch?v=foehpsv-2TE

LOW-HISTAMINE DIET
- The Swiss Interest Group Histamine Intolerance site, which contains a list of low-histamine and high-histamine foods: https://www.mastzellaktivierung.info

References

- Lawrence Afrin, Mary Ackerley, Linda Bluestein, et al. Diagnosis of mast cell activation syndrome: a global 'consensus-2'. *Diagnosis* 2020; 8: 137–52.
- AgelessRx. Pilot study into LDN and NAD+ for treatment of patients with post-COVID-19 syndrome. *ClinicalTrials. gov*, 27 October 2020. Available at https://clinicaltrials.gov/ct2/show/NCT04604704
- Gustavo Aguirre-Chang, Eduardo C Saavedra, Maneul Yui, et al. Post-acute or prolonged COVID-19: ivermectin treatment for patients with persistent symptoms. *Zenodo* (preprint) 2020. DOI:10.5281/zenodo.4058612.
- Hayder M Al-kuraishy, Ali I Al-Gareeb, Safaa Qusti, et al. Covid-19-induced dysautonomia: a menace of sympathetic storm. *American Society for Neurochemistry* 2021; 13: 1–10.
- Danny M Altmann, Rosemary J Boyton. Decoding the unknowns in Long Covid. *British Medical Journal* 2021; 372: n132.
- Sarah J Annesley, Paul R Fisher. Lymphoblastoid cell lines as models to study mitochondrial function in neurological disorders. *International Journal of Molecular Science* 2021; 22: 4536.
- Dalia Arostegui, Kenny Castro, Steven Schwarz Vaidy, et al. Persistent SARS-CoV-2 nucleocapsid protein presence in the intestinal epithelium of a pediatric patient 3 months after acute infection. *Journal of Pediatric Gastroenterology and Nutrition Reports* 2022; 3: e152.
- M S Arruda, C A Petta, M S Abrao, et al. Time elapsed from onset of symptoms to diagnosis of endometriosis in a cohort study of Brazilian women. *Human Reproduction* 2003; 18: 756–59.

- L Attademo, F Bernardini. Are dopamine and serotonin involved in COVID-19 pathophysiology? *European Journal of Psychiatry* 2021; 35: 62–63.
- Axcella. AXA1125 now in phase 2a and 2b development. Axcella, 13 June 2022. Available at https://axcellatx.com/pipeline/axa1125/
- Daniel Ayoubkhani, Charlotte Bermingham, Koen B Pouwels, et al. Trajectory of Long Covid symptoms after Covid-19 vaccination: community-based cohort study. *BMJ* 2022; 377: e069676.
- Henry H Balfour, Oludare A Odumade, David O Schmeling, et al. Behavioral, virologic, and immunologic factors associated with acquisition and severity of primary Epstein-Barr virus infection in university students. *Journal of Infectious Diseases* 2013; 207: 80–88.
- Tessa J Barrett, Macintosh Cornwell, Khrystyna Myndzar, et al. Platelets amplify endotheliopathy in COVID-19. *Science Advances* 2021; 7: eabh2434.
- Paul Bastard, Lindsey B Rosen, Qian Zhang, et al. Autoantibodies against type I IFNs in patients with life-threatening COVID-19. *Science* 2020; 370: eabd4585.
- Kjetil Bjornevik, Marianna Cortese, Brian C Healy. Longitudinal analysis reveals high prevalence of Epstein-Barr virus associated with multiple sclerosis. *Science* 2022; 375: 296–301.
- Monica J Bolton, Bryan P Chapman, Harm Van Marwijk. Low-dose naltrexone as a treatment for chronic fatigue syndrome. *BMJ Case Reports* 2020; 13: e232502.
- Stefan R Bornstein, Karin Voit-Bak, Timo Donate, et al. Chronic post-COVID-19 syndrome and chronic fatigue syndrome: is there a role for extracorporeal apheresis? *Molecular Psychiatry* 2022; 27: 34–37.
- Kinga P Böszörményi, Marieke A Stammes, Zarah C Fagrouch, et al. The post-acute phase of SARS-CoV-2 infection in two macaque species is associated with signs of ongoing

virus replication and pathology in pulmonary and extrapulmonary tissues. *Viruses* 2021; 13: 1673.

- Harry Brown. Ten most common conditions seen by GPs. *British Journal of Family Medicine*, 8 July 2019. Available at https://www.bjfm.co.uk/ten-most-common-conditions-seen-by-gps

- Gaetano Bulfamante, Tommaso Bocci, Monica Falleni, et al. Brainstem neuropathology in two cases of COVID-19: SARS-CoV-2 trafficking between brain and lung. *Journal of Neurology* 2021; 268: 4486–91.

- Dave Burke, Neil Shaw. Tillie, 11, still has a feeding tube a year after catching COVID. *WalesOnline*, 1 February 2022. Available at https://www.walesonline.co.uk/news/uk-news/tillie-11-still-feeding-tube-22941350

- Carlo Cervia, Yves Zurbuchen, Patrick Taeschler, et al. Immunoglobulin signature predicts risk of post-acute COVID-19 syndrome. *Nature Communications* 2022; 13: 446.

- S Charfeddine, H I Jadjamor, S Torjmen, et al. Sulodexide in the treatment of patients with long COVID 19 symptoms and endothelial dysfunction: the results of TUN-EndCOV study. *Archives of Cardiovascular Diseases Supplements* 2022; 14: 127.

- Daniel Chertow, Sydney Stein, Sabrina Ramelli, et al. SARS-CoV-2 infection and persistence throughout the human body and brain. *Research Square* (preprint) 2022. DOI:10.21203/rs.3.rs-1139035/v1.

- Anushal Chidharla, Salman B Syed, Tulika Chatterjee, et al. A case report of COVID-associated catastrophic antiphospholipid syndrome successfully treated with eculizumab. *Journal of Blood Medicine* 2021; 12: 929–33.

- Jan Choutka, Viraj Jansari, Mady Hornig, et al. Unexplained post-acute infection syndromes. *Nature Medicine* 2022; 28: 911–23.

- Ernest Choy, Serge Perrot, Teresa Leon, et al. A patient survey of the impact of fibromyalgia and the journey to diagnosis. *BMC Health Services Research* 2010; 10: 102.

- Plinio Cirillo, Vittirio Taglialatela, Grazia Pellegrino, et al. Effects of colchicine on platelet aggregation in patients on dual antiplatelet therapy with aspirin and clopidogrel. *Journal of Thrombosis and Thrombolysis* 2020; 50: 468–72.

- Simon M Collin, Inger J Bakken, Irwin Nazareth, et al. Trends in the incidence of chronic fatigue syndrome and fibromyalgia in the UK, 2001–2013: a Clinical Practice Research Datalink study. *Journal of the Royal Society of Medicine* 2017; 110: 231–44.

- Esther M Crawley, Daisy M Gaunt, Kirsty Garfield, et al. Clinical and cost-effectiveness of the Lightning Process in addition to specialist medical care for paediatric chronic fatigue syndrome: randomised controlled trial. *Archives of Disease in Childhood* 2018; 103: 155–64.

- Carolyn Crist. More than 100 million people worldwide have or had Long COVID: study. *WebMD*, 18 November 2021. Available at https://www.webmd.com/lung/news/20211118/millions-worldwide-long-covid-study

- Melanie Dani, Andreas Dirksen, Patricia Taraborrelli, et al. Autonomic dysfunction in 'Long COVID': rationale, physiology and management strategies. *Clinical Medicine* 2021; 21: e63–67.

- Hannah E Davis, Gina S Assaf, Lisa McCorkell, et al. Characterising long COVID in an international cohort: 7 months of symptoms and their impact. *eClinicalMedicine* 2021; 38: 101019.

- Luiz G F de Assis Barros D'Elia Zanella and Luciana de Lima Galvão. The COVID-19 burden or tryptophan syndrome: autoimmunity, immunoparalysis and tolerance in a tumorigenic environment. *Journal of Infectious Diseases and Epidemiology* 2021; 7: 195.

- Andrea Dennis, Malgorzata Wamil, Johann Alberts, et al. Multiorgan impairment in low-risk individuals with post-COVID-19 syndrome: a prospective, community-based study. *BMJ Open* 2022; 11: e048391.

- Guilherme Dias De Melo, Françoise Lazarine, Sylvain Levallois, et al. COVID-19-related anosmia is associated with viral persistence and inflammation in human olfactory epithelium and brain infection in hamsters. *Science Translational Medicine* 2021; 13: eabf8396.
- Joel E Dimsdale. Psychological stress and cardiovascular disease. *Journal of the American College of Cardiology* 2008; 51: 1237–46.
- Gwenaëlle Douaud, Soojin Lee, Fidel Alfaro-Almagro, et al. SARS-CoV-2 is associated with changes in brain structure in UK Biobank. *Nature* 2022; 604: 697–707.
- DrugBank Online. Zofin. DrugBank Online, 13 June 2022. Available at https://go.drugbank.com/drugs/DB16519.
- Karin Due Bruun, Kirstine Amris, Henrik B Vagter, et al. Low-dose naltrexone for the treatment of fibromyalgia: protocol for a double-blind, randomized, placebo-controlled trial. *Trials* 2021; 22: 804.
- Maya Dusenberry. *Doing Harm: The Truth About How Bad Medicine and Lazy Science Leave Women Dismissed, Misdiagnosed, and Sick.* London: HarperOne, 2017.
- Jessica A Eccles, Beth Thompson, Kristy Themelis, et al. Beyond bones: the relevance of variants of connective tissue (hypermobility) to fibromyalgia, ME/CFS and controversies surrounding diagnostic classification: an observational study. *Clinical Medicine* 2021; 21: 53–58.
- Jonathan C W Edwards, Simon McGrath, Adrian Baldwin, et al. The biological challenge of myalgic encephalomyelitis/chronic fatigue syndrome: a solvable problem. *Fatigue* 2016; 4: 63–69.
- Endometriosis UK. Endometriosis facts and figures. Endometriosis UK, 2022. Available at https://www.endometriosis-uk.org/endometriosis-facts-and-figures
- İmdat Eroğlu, Burcu Çelik Eroğlu, Gülay Sain Güven. Altered tryptophan absorption and metabolism could

underlie long-term symptoms in survivors of coronavirus disease 2019 (COVID-19). *Nutrition* 2021; 90: 111308.

- Experimental Biology. Study shows dogs can accurately sniff out cancer in blood. *Science Daily*, 8 April 2019. Available at sciencedaily.com/releases/2019/04/190408114304.htm.
- Anthony Fernández-Castañeda, Peiwen Lu, Anna C Geraghty, et al. Mild respiratory SARS-CoV-2 infection can cause multi-lineage cellular dysregulation and myelin loss in the brain. *bioRxiv* (preprint) 2022. DOI:10.1101/2022.0 1.07.475453.
- Markus Feuerer, Laura Herrero, Daniela Cipolletta, et al. Fat T_{reg} cells: a liaison between the immune and metabolic systems. *Nature Medicine* 2009; 15: 930–39.
- Christian Gaebler, Zijun Wang, Julio C Lorenzi, et al. Evolution of antibody immunity to SARS-CoV-2. *Nature* 2021; 591: 639–44.
- Paul Garner. Covid-19 at 14 weeks–phantom speed cameras, unknown limits, and harsh penalties. *BMJ Opinion*, 23 June 2020. Available at https://blogs.bmj.com/bmj/2020/06/23/paul-garner-covid-19-at-14-weeks-phantom-speed-cameras-unknown-limits-and-harsh-penalties/
- Naama Geva-Zatorsky, Esen Sefik, Lindsay Kua, et al. Mining the human gut microbiota for immunomodulatory organisms. *Resource* 2017; 168: 928–43.
- Ronald Glaser, Janice Kiecolt-Glaser. Stress-induced immune dysfunction: implications for health. *Nature Reviews Immunology* 2005; 5: 243–51.
- Danielle Glick, Sandra Barth, Kay F Macleod. Autophagy: cellular and molecular mechanisms. *The Journal of Pathology* 2010; 221: 3–12.
- Paul Glynne, Natasha Tahmasedi, Vanya Grant, et al. Long COVID following mild SARS-CoV-2 infection: characteristic T cell alterations and response to antihistamines. *Journal of Investigative Medicine* 2022; 70: 61–67.

- Denise Goh, Jeffrey C Lim, Sonia B Fernandez, et al. Persistence of residual SARS-CoV-2 viral antigen and RNA in tissues of patients with Long COVID-19. *Research Square* (preprint) 2022. DOI:10.21203/rs.3.rs-1379777/v1.
- Dominique Grandjean, Dominique Salmon, Dorsaf Slama, et al. Screening for SARS-CoV-2 persistence in Long COVID patients using sniffer dogs and scents from axillary sweats samples. *Journal of Clinical Trials* 2021; 12: 1000002.
- James T Grist, Guilhem J Collier, Huw Walters, et al. The investigation of pulmonary abnormalities using hyperpolarised xenon magnetic resonance imaging in patients with long-COVID. *medRxiv* (preprint) 2022. DOI:10.1101/2022.02.01.22269999.
- Lize M Grobbelaar, Chantelle Venter, Mare Vlok, et al. SARS-CoV-2 spike protein S1 induces fibrin(ogen) resistant to fibrinolysis: implications for microclot formation in COVID-19. *Bioscience Reports* 2021; 41: BSR20210611.
- Benjamin Groth, Padmaja Venkatakrishnan, Su-Ju Lin. NAD+ metabolism, metabolic stress, and infection. *Frontiers in Molecular Biosciences* 2021; 8: 686412.
- E Guedj, J Y Campion, P Dudouet, et al. 18F-FDG brain PET hypometabolism in patients with long COVID. *European Journal of Nuclear Medicine and Molecular Imaging* 2021; 48: 2823–83.
- Deepthi Gurdasani, Athena Akrami, Valerie C Bradley, et al. Long COVID in children. *The Lancet Child & Adolescent Health* 2022; 6: e2.
- Britta Haenisch, Markus M Nöthen, Gerhard J Molderings. Systemic mast cell activation disease: the role of molecular genetic alterations in pathogenesis, heritability and diagnostics. *Immunology* 2012; 137: 197–205.
- Asa Hakansson, Goran Molin. Gut microbiota and inflammation. *Nutrients* 2011; 3: 637–82.

- Heidi L Heard, Marsha M Linehan. Dialectical behavior therapy: an integrative approach to the treatment of borderline personality disorder. *Journal of Psychotherapy Integration* 1994; 4: 55–82.
- Paul M Heerdt, Ben Shelley, Inderjit Singh. Impaired systemic oxygen extraction long after mild COVID-19: potential perioperative implications. *British Journal of Anaesthesia* 2022; 128: e246–49.
- Nadine Herr, Chirstophe Bode, Daniel Duerschmied. The effects of serotonin in immune cells. *Frontiers in Cardiovascular Medicine* 2017; 4: 48.
- Sammy Heung. Hong Kong team develops test for long Covid so recovered patients can tell if trouble lies ahead. *South China Morning Post*, 11 April 2022. Available at https://www.scmp.com/news/hong-kong/health-environment/article/3173759/hong-kong-team-develops-test-long-covid-so.
- Marisa E Hilliard, Joyce P Yi-Frazier, Danielle Hessler, et al. Stress and A1c among people with diabetes across the lifespan. *Current Diabetes Reports* 2016; 16: 67.
- Chanawee Hirunpattarasilp, Gregory James, Felipe Freitas, et al. SARS-CoV-2 binding to ACE2 triggers pericyte-mediated angiotensin-evoked cerebral capillary constriction. *bioRxiv* (preprint) 2021. DOI:10.1101/2021.04.01.438122.
- Sean Holden, Rebekah Maksoud, Natalie Eaton-Fitch, et al. A systematic review of mitochondrial abnormalities in myalgic encephalomyelitis/chronic fatigue syndrome/systemic exertion intolerance disease. *Journal of Translational Medicine* b; 18: 290.
- Erin Hopkins, Terrence Sanvictores, Sandeep Sharma. Physiology, acid base balance. *StatPearls*, 14 September 2021. Available at https://www.ncbi.nlm.nih.gov/books/NBK507807/
- Juul Houwen, Peter L B J Lucassen, Hugo W Stappers, et al. Medically unexplained symptoms: time to and triggers

for diagnosis in primary care consultations. *British Journal of General Practice* 2020; 70: e86–94.

- Dan Hurley. Sleep neurologists call it 'COVID-somnia'– increased sleep disturbances linked to the pandemic. *NeurologyToday*, 9 July 2020. Available at https://journals.lww.com/neurotodayonline/fulltext/2020/07090/sleep_neurologists_call_it.1.aspx

- Institute of Medicine of the National Academies. *Beyond Myalgic Encephalomyelitis/Chronic Fatigue Syndrome: Redefining an Illness*. Washington, DC: The National Academies Press, 2015.

- Elizabeth Iveson. Feasibility of cannabidiol for the treatment of Long COVID. *ClinicalTrials.gov*, 13 June 2022. Available at https://clinicaltrials.gov/ct2/show/NCT04997395

- Laura Jefferson, Karen Bloor, Alan Maynard. Women in medicine: historical perspectives and recent trends. *British Medical Bulletin* 2015; 114: 5–15.

- Cort Johnson. Berlin Cures … ? Could BC 007 help with Long COVID and ME/CFS? *Health Rising*, 30 December 2021. Available at https://www.healthrising.org/blog/2021/12/30/bc-007-berlin-cures-long-covid-chronic-fatigue-syndrome/

- Shane Kelly, Noel Pollock, George Polglass, et al. Injury and illness in elite athletics: a prospective cohort study over three seasons. *International Journal of Sports Physical Therapy* 2022; 17: 420–33.

- Ritsuko Kohno, David S Cannom, Brian Olshansky et al. Mast cell activation disorder and postural orthostatic tachycardia syndrome: a clinical association. *Journal of the American Heart Association* 2021; 10: e021002.

- Krister Kristensson, Erling Norrby. Persistence of RNA viruses in the central nervous system. *Annual Review of Microbiology* 1986; 40: 159–84.

- Jason Laday. More than 50% of patients with COVID-19 positive for antiphospholipid antibodies. *Healio*,

8 November 2020. Available at https://www.healio.com/ news/rheumatology/20201108/more-than-50-of-patients-with-covid19-positive-for-antiphospholipid-antibodies

- J S Lawrence, V A Laine, R de Graaff. The epidemiology of rheumatoid arthritis in northern Europe. *Proceedings of the Royal Society of Medicine* 1961; 54: 454–62.

- Luke D Liu, Deborah L Duricka. Stellate ganglion block reduces symptoms of Long COVID: a case series. *Journal of Neuroimmunology* 2022; 362: 577784.

- Cristina Lluch, Laura Galiana, Pablo Domenech, et al. The impact of the COVID-19 pandemic on burnout, compassion fatigue, and compassion satisfaction in healthcare personnel: a systematic review of the literature published during the first year of the pandemic. *Healthcare* 2022; 10: 364.

- Sandra Lopez-Leon, Talia Wegman-Ostrosky, Carol Perelman, et al. More than 50 long-term effects of COVID-19: a systematic review and meta-analysis. *Nature* 2021; 11: 16144.

- Sandra Lopez-Leon, Talia Wegman-Ostrosky, Cipatli Ayuzo del Valle, et al. Long-COVID in children and adolescents: a systematic review and meta-analyses. *medRxiv* (preprint) 2022. DOI:10.1101/2022.03.10.22272237.

- Frances McGarry, John Gow, Peter O Behan. Enterovirus in the chronic fatigue syndrome. *Annals of Internal Medicine* 1994; 120: 972–73.

- Ross McGuinness. How many children have actually had COVID? *Yahoo! News*, 12 November 2021. Available at https://uk.news.yahoo.com/how-many-children-covid-coronavirus-165555811.html

- Angus Mackay. A paradigm for post-Covid-19 fatigue syndrome analogous to ME/CFS. *Frontiers in Neurology* 2021; 12: 701419.

- Robin McKie. Only 29% of UK COVID hospital patients recover within a year. *The Guardian*, 24 April 2022. Available at https://www.theguardian.com/world/2022/

apr/24/only-29-of-uk-covid-hospital-patients-recover-within-a-year

- Elisabeth Mahase. Covid-19: Pfizer's paxlovid is 89% effective in patients at risk of serious illness, company reports. *British Medical Journal* 2021; 375: n2713.
- Laura Maintz, Natalija Novak. Histamine and histamine intolerance. *The American Journal of Clinical Nutrition* 2007; 85: 1185–96.
- Albert Martin-Cardona, Josep Lloreta Trull, Raquel Albero-González, et al. SARS-CoV-2 identified by transmission electron microscopy in lymphoproliferative and ischaemic intestinal lesions of COVID-19 patients with acute abdominal pain: two case reports. *BMC Gastroenterology* 2021; 21: 334.
- Arthur Melkumyants, Ludmila Buryachkovskaya, Nikita Lomakin. Mild COVID-19 and impaired blood cell–endothelial crosstalk: considering long-term use of antithrombotics? *Thrombosis and Haemostasis* 2022; 122: 123–30.
- Pierre L Meroni, Maria O Borghi. Antiphospholipid antibodies and COVID-19 thrombotic vasculopathy: one swallow does not make a summer. *Annals of the Rheumatic Diseases* 2021; 80: 1105–07.
- R Miller, A R Wentzel, G A Richards. COVID-19: NAD+ deficiency may predispose the aged, obese and type 2 diabetics to mortality through its effect on SIRT1 activity. *Medical Hypotheses* 2020; 144: 110044.
- Christine Miserandino. The spoon theory. *ButYouDon'tLookSick*, 2003. Available at https://butyoudontlooksick.com/articles/written-by-christine/the-spoon-theory/
- Daniel Missailidis, Sarah J Annesley, Claire Y Allan, et al. An isolated complex V inefficiency and dysregulated mitochondrial function in immortalized lymphocytes

from ME/CFS patients. *International Journal of Molecular Science* 2020; 21: 1074.

- Maria Ines Mitrani, Michael A Bellio, Allen Meglin, et al. Treatment of a COVID-19 long hauler with an amniotic fluid-derived extracellular vesicle biologic. *Respir Med Case Rep* 2021; 34: 101502.

- Harvey Moldofsky, John Patcai. Chronic widespread musculoskeletal pain, fatigue, depression and disordered sleep in chronic post-SARS syndrome; a case-controlled study. *BMC Neurology* 2011; 11: 37.

- Erika Molteni, Carole H Sudre, Liane S Canas, et al. Illness duration and symptom profile in symptomatic UK school-aged children tested for SARS-CoV-2. *The Lancet Child & Adolescent Health* 2021; 5: 708–18.

- Valeria Mondelli, Carmine Pariante. What can neuroimmunology teach us about the symptoms of long-COVID? *Oxford Open Immunology* 2021; 2: iqab004.

- Gerwyn Morris, George Anderson, Michael Maes. Hypothalamic-pituitary-adrenal hypofunction in myalgic encephalomyelitis (ME)/chronic fatigue syndrome (CFS) as a consequence of activated immune-inflammatory and oxidative and nitrosative pathways. *Molecular Neurobiology* 2016; 54: 6806–19.

- Kellen Mulhern. 1261 the long term exhaustion of a viral infection. *Sleep* 2021; 43: A480.

- Aravind Natarajan, Sumaya Zlitni, Erin F Brooks, et al. Gastrointestinal symptoms and fecal shedding of SARS-CoV-2 RNA suggest prolonged gastrointestinal infection. *Med* 2022. DOI:10.1016/j.medj.2022.04.001.

- National Institute for Health and Care Excellence. Rheumatoid arthritis: how common is it? National Institute for Health and Care Excellence, 2020. Available at https://cks.nice.org.uk/topics/rheumatoid-arthritis/background-information/prevalence-incidence/

- National Institute for Health and Care Excellence. Nicotinic acid. *British National Formulary* 13 June 2022. Available at https://bnf.nice.org.uk/drug/nicotinic-acid.html
- National Institutes of Health. NIH launches new initiative to study 'Long COVID'. National Institutes of Health, 23 February 2021. Available at https://www.nih.gov/about-nih/who-we-are/nih-director/statements/nih-launches-new-initiative-study-long-covid
- Jenny C Ngai, Fanny W Ko, Susanna S Ng, et al. The long-term impact of severe acute respiratory syndrome on pulmonary function, exercise capacity and health status. *Respirology* 2010; 15: 543–50.
- Peter Novak, Shibani S Mukerji, Haitham S Alabsi, et al. Multisystem involvement in post-acute sequelae of coronavirus disease 19. *Annals of Neurology* 2022; 91: 367–79.
- Martine Nurek, Clare Rayner, Anette Freyer, et al. Recommendations for the recognition, diagnosis, and management of long COVID: a Delphi study. *British Journal of General Practice* 2021; 71: e815–20.
- Aoife O'Donovan, Beth E Cohen, Karen H Seal, et al. Elevated risk for autoimmune disorders in Iraq and Afghanistan veterans with posttraumatic stress disorder. *Biological Psychiatry* 2015; 77: 365–74.
- Aoife O'Donovan, Beth E Cohen, Karen H Seal, et al. Elevated risk for autoimmune disorders in Iraq and Afghanistan veterans with posttraumatic stress disorder. *Biological Psychiatry* 2015; 77: 365–74.
- Office for National Statistics. Prevalence of ongoing symptoms following coronavirus (COVID-19) infection in the UK: 1 June 2022. Office for National Statistics, 1 June 2022. Available at https://www.ons.gov.uk/peoplepopulationandcommunity/healthandsocialcare/conditionsanddiseases/bulletins/prevalenceofongoingsymptomsfollowingcoronaviruscovid19infectionintheuk/1june2022

- Evangelos Oikonomou, Nektarios Souvaliotis, Stamatios Lampsas, et al. Endothelial dysfunction in acute and long standing COVID-19: A prospective cohort study. *Vascular Pharmacology*; 2022; 144: 106975.
- David Olson, Lisa S Colangelo. Doctors struggle to find answers for children with Long Covid. Newsday, 4 April 2022. Available at https://www.newsday.com/news/health/coronavirus/long-covid-in-kids-cndfs9p1
- Organicell Regenerative Medicine. Zofin to treat COVID-19 long haulers. *ClinicalTrials.gov*, 14 April 2022. Available at https://clinicaltrials.gov/ct2/show/NCT05228899
- Páraic S O'Súilleabháin, Nicholas A Turiano, Denis Gerstorf, et al. Personality pathways to mortality: Interleukin-6 links conscientiousness to mortality risk. *Brain, Behaviour & Immunity* 2021; 93: 238–44.
- Oliver O'Sullivan. Long-term sequelae following previous coronavirus epidemics. *Clinical Medicine* 2021; 68–70.
- Kezia Parkins. Resolve Therapeutics to start phase II trial of RSLV-132 for long Covid. *Clinical Trials Arena*, 24 June 2021. Available at https://www.clinicaltrialsarena.com/news/resolve-therapeutics-to-start-phase-ii-trial-of-rslv-132-for-long-covid/
- John Patcai. Is 'Long Covid' similar to 'Long SARS'? *Oxford Open Immunology* 2022; 3: iqac002.
- Bruce K Patterson, Edgar B Francisco, Ram Yogendra, et al. Persistence of SARS CoV-2 S1 protein in CD16+ monocytes in post-acute sequelae of COVID-19 (PASC) up to 15 months post-infection. *Frontiers in Immunology* 2022; 12: 746021.
- Bruce K Patterson, Jose Guevara-Coto, Ram Yogendra, et al. Immune-based prediction of COVID-19 severity and chronicity decoded using machine learning. *Frontiers in Immunology* 2021; 12: 700782.

- Bruce Patterson, Ram Yogendra, José Guevara-Coto, et al. Targeting the monocytic-endothelial-platelet axis with maraviroc and pravastatin as a therapeutic option to treat Long COVID/ post-acute sequelae of COVID (PASC). *Research Square* (preprint) 2022. DOI:10.21203/rs.3.rs-1344323/ v1.

- Amanda B Payne, Zunera Gilani, Shana Godfred-Cato, et al. Incidence of multisystem inflammatory syndrome in children among US persons infected with SARS-CoV-2. *JAMA Network Open* 2021; 4; e2116420.

- Neil Pearce, Juha Pekkanen, Richard Beasley. How much asthma is really attributable to atopy? *Thorax* 1999; 54: 268–72.

- Stephen W Porges. The polyvagal theory: new insights into adaptive reactions of the autonomic nervous system. *Cleveland Clinic Journal of Medicine* 2009; 76: 86–90.

- PoTS UK. GP guide: PoTS on a page. PoTS, 2022. Available at https://www.potsuk.org/pots-for-medics/gp-guide/

- Andrea Pozzi. COVID-19 and mitochondrial non-coding RNAs: new insights from published data. *Frontiers in Physiology* 2022; 12: 805005.

- Etheresia Pretorius, Chantelle Venter, Gert J Laubscher, et al. Combined triple treatment of fibrin amyloid microclots and platelet pathology in individuals with long COVID/ post-acute sequelae of COVID-19 (PASC) can resolve their persistent symptoms. *Research Square* (preprint) 2022. DOI:10.21203/rs.3.rs-1205453/v2.

- Etheresia Pretorius, Mare Vlok, Chantelle Venter, et al. Persistent clotting protein pathology in long COVID/ post-acute sequelae of COVID-19 (PASC) is accompanied by increased levels of antiplasmin. *Cardiovascular Diabetology* 2021; 20: 172.

- PREVAIL III Study Group. A longitudinal study of Ebola sequelae in Liberia. *New England Journal of Medicine* 2019; 380: 924–34.

- Amy D Proal, Michael B VanElzakker. Long COVID or post-acute sequelae of COVID-19 (PASC): an overview of biological factors that may contribute to persistent symptoms. *Frontiers in Microbiology* 2021; 12: 698169.
- Yuanyuan Qin, Jinfeng Wu, Tao Chen, et al. Long-term microstructure and cerebral blood flow changes in patients recovered from COVID-19 without neurological manifestations. *The Journal of Clinical Investigation* 2021; 131: e147329.
- R K Rao, G Samak. Protection and restitution of gut barrier by probiotics: nutritional and clinical implications. *Current Nutrition and Food Science* 2013; 9: 99–107.
- RCSI. Blood clotting may be the root cause of Long COVID syndrome, research shows. *Science Daily*, 16 August 2021. Available at https://www.sciencedaily.com/releases/2021/08/210816125717.htm
- Thibault Renoir, Kyoko Hasebe, Laura Gray. Mind and body: how the health of the body impacts on neuropsychiatry. *Frontiers in Pharmacology* 2013; 4: 158.
- Resolve Therapeutics. Phase 2 study of RSLV-132 in subjects with long COVID. *ClinicalTrials.gov*, 25 June 2021. Available at https://clinicaltrials.gov/ct2/show/NCT04944121
- Guy A Richards, Adrian Wentzel, Robert Miller, et al. Post-acute COVID-19 sequelae – 'COVID long hauler'. *Wits Journal of Clinical Medicine* 2021; 3: 117–24.
- Tim Robbins, Michael Gonevski, Cain Clark, et al. Hyperbaric oxygen therapy for the treatment of long COVID: early evaluation of a highly promising intervention. *Clinical Medicine* 2021; 21: e629–32.
- Jessica S Rogers-Brown, Valentine Wanga, Catherine Okoro, et al. Outcomes among patients referred to outpatient rehabilitation clinics after COVID-19 diagnosis – United States, January 2020–March 2021. *Morbidity and Mortality Weekly Report* 2021; 70: 967–71.

- Gez Medinger. Can symptoms alone diagnose COVID-19? / Comprehensive symptom studies analysis. 9 July 2020. Available at https://www.youtube.com/watch?v=24IJ2dHbYPk
- Gez Medinger. Who gets Long Covid, and why? | Huge findings from new study. 6 November 2020. Available at https://www.youtube.com/watch?v=hnPvw20iH80&ab_channel=RUN-DMC%2FGezMedinger
- Gez Medinger. Here's how you treat Long Covid | Lessons from MCAS – Dr Tina Peers. 24 November 2020. Available at https://www.youtube.com/watch?v=sICD0Kn6pR4
- Gez Medinger. First effective treatment for Long Covid | Stunning data from huge new study. 22 December 2020. Available at https://www.youtube.com/watch?v=9-3V3honcIA
- Gez Medinger. Long Covid: one year in | How many have recovered? Comprehensive new study analysed. 2 April 2021. Available at https://www.youtube.com/watch?v=Ox1c10VsQoM
- Gez Medinger. Long Covid at 18 months | How many have recovered – and what's their secret? 25 October 2021. Available at https://www.youtube.com/watch?v=cKreDsa_GqM
- Gez Medinger. The Great experiment: can activity play a role in Long Covid recovery? 19 January 2022. Available at https://www.youtube.com/watch?v=UCJhYAQ6aGk
- Gez Medinger. The puzzle comes together – why dysfunctional metabolism might explain Long Covid. 13 February 2022. Available at https://www.youtube.com/watch?v=ZFPleh6z7io
- Gez Medinger. Long Covid at two years: how many have recovered? 13 May 2022. Available at https://www.youtube.com/watch?v=aJokJnBLOMw

- Feargal J Ryan, Christopher M Hope, Makutiro G Masavuli, et al. Long-term perturbation of the peripheral immune system months after SARS-CoV-2 infection. *BMC Medicine* 2022; 20: 26.
- Corinna Sadlier, Werner C Albrich, Ujjwal Neogi, et al. Metabolic rewiring and serotonin depletion in patients with postacute sequelae of COVID-19. *Allergy* 2022; 77: 1623–25.
- Joshua D Safer, Eli Coleman, Jamie Feldman, et al. Barriers to health care for transgender individuals. *Current Opinion in Endocrinology, Diabetes & Obesity* 2016; 23: 168–71.
- Juan P Sanabria-Mazo, Jesus Montero-Marin, Albert Feliu-Soler, et al. Mindfulness-based program plus amygdala and insula retraining (MAIR) for the treatment of women with fibromyalgia: a pilot randomized controlled trial. *Journal of Clinical Medicine* 2020; 9: 3246.
- Carolina X Sandler, Vegard B Wyller, Rona Moss-Morris, et al. Long COVID and post-infective fatigue syndrome: a review. *Open Forum Infectious Diseases* 2021; 8: 440.
- Tania M V Santos, Ana M Pereira, Reginaldo G C Lopes, et al. Lag time between onset of symptoms and diagnosis of endometriosis. *Einstein* 2012; 10: 39–43.
- Bernadette Schurink, Eva Roos, Teadora Radonic, et al. Viral presence and immunopathology in patients with lethal COVID-19: a prospective autopsy cohort study. *The Lancet Microbe* 2020; 1: e290–99.
- Emilia Sforza, David Hupin, Frédéric Roche. Mononucleosis: a possible cause of idiopathic hypersomnia. *Frontiers in Neurology* 2018; 9: 922.
- Xu-Rui Shen, Rong Geng, Qian Li, et al. ACE2-independent infection of T lymphocytes by SARS-CoV-2. *Signal Transduction and Targeted Therapy* 2022; 7: 83.
- Jonathan E Sherin. Post-traumatic stress disorder: the neurobiological impact of psychological trauma. *Dialogues in Clinical Neuroscience* 2011; 13: 263–78.

- Inderjit Singh, Phillip Joseph, Paul M Heerdt, et al. Persistent exertional intolerance after COVID-19: insights from invasive cardiopulmonary exercise testing. *Chest* 2022; 161: 54–63.
- Yuji Soejima, Takao Munemoto, Akinori Masuda, et al. Effects of Waon therapy on chronic fatigue syndrome: a pilot study. *Internal Medicine* 2015; 53: 333–38.
- Ahmed M Soliman, Mahesh Fuldeore, Michael C Snabes. Factors associated with time to endometriosis diagnosis in the United States. *Journal of Women's Health* 2017; 26: 788–97.
- Eric Song, Christopher M Bartley, Ryan D Chow, et al. Divergent and self-reactive immune responses in the CNS of COVID-19 patients with neurological symptoms. *Cell Reports Medicine* 2021; 2: 100288.
- Huan Song, Fang Fang, Gunnar Tomasson, et al. Association of stress-related disorders with subsequent autoimmune disease. *Journal of the American Medical Association* 2018; 319: 2388–400.
- STIMULATE-ICP. About the STIMULATE-ICP study. STIMULATE-ICP, 2022. Available at https://www.stimulate-icp.org/about
- Yapeng Su, Dan Yuan, Daniel G Chen, et al. Multiple early factors anticipate post-acute COVID-19 sequelae. *Cell* 2022; 185: 881–95.
- Carole H Sudre, Benjamin Murray, Thomas Varsavsky, et al. Attributes and predictors of long COVID. *Nature Medicine* 2021; 27: 626–31.
- Weiguo Sun, Linxia Zhang, Lejian Lin, et al. Chronic psychological stress impairs germinal center response by repressing miR-155. *Brain, Behaviour & Immunity* 2019; 76: 48–60.
- Zoe Swank, Yasmeen Senussi, Galit Alter, et al. Persistent circulating SARS-CoV-2 spike is associated with post-acute COVID-19 sequelae. *medRxiv* (preprint) 2022. DOI:10.1101/2022.06.14.22276401.

- Maxime Taquet, Quentin Dercon, Sierra Luciano, et al. Incidence, co-occurrence, and evolution of long-COVID features: a 6 month retrospective cohort study of 273,618 survivors of COVID-19. *PLoS Medicine* 2021; 18: e1003773.
- Francisco Tejerina, Pilar Catalan, Cristina Rodriguez-Grande, et al. Post-COVID-19 syndrome. SARS-CoV-2 RNA detection in plasma, stool, and urine in patients with persistent symptoms after COVID-19. *BMC Infectious Diseases* 2022; 22: 211.
- Elden Berla Thangam, Ebenezer Angel Jemima, Himadri Singh, et al. The role of histamine and histamine receptors in mast cell-mediated allergy and inflammation: the hunt for new therapeutic targets. *Frontiers in Immunology* 2018; 9: 1873.
- Robert Thomas, Madeline Williams, Jeffrey Aldous, et al. A randomised, double-blind, placebo-controlled trial evaluating concentrated phytochemical-rich nutritional capsule in addition to a probiotic capsule on clinical outcomes among individuals with COVID-19–the UK Phyto-V Study. *COVID* 2022; 2: 433–49.
- Ingrid Torjesen. Pressure grows on *Lancet* to review 'flawed' PACE trial. *British Medical Journal* 2018; 362: k3621.
- Viet-Thi Tran, Raphaël Porcher, Isabelle Pane, et al. Course of post COVID-19 disease symptoms over time in the ComPaRe Long COVID prospective e-cohort. *Nature Communications* 2022; 13: 1812.
- David Tuller. Trial by error: the troubling case of the PACE chronic fatigue syndrome study. *Virology Blog*, 21 October 2015. Available at https://www.virology.ws/2015/10/21/trial-by-error-i/
- University of Oxford. New research studies to help diagnose and treat Long COVID funded by NIHR. University of Oxford, 19 July 2021. Available at https://www.ox.ac.uk/news/2021–07-19-new-research-studies-help-diagnose-and-treat-long-covid-funded-nihr

- Bessel van der Kolk. *The Body Keeps the Score: Mind, Brain and Body in the Transformation of Trauma.* London: Penguin Books, 2015.
- Alyssa N Varanoske, Holly L McClung, John J Sepowitz, et al. Stress and the gut-brain axis: cognitive performance, mood state, and biomarkers of blood-brain barrier and intestinal permeability following severe physical and psychological stress. *Brain, Behaviour & Immunity* 2022; 101: 383–93.
- Luigi Vimercati, Luigi De Maria, Marco Quarato, et al. Association between Long Covid and overweight/obesity. *Clinical Medicine* 2021; 10: 4143.
- Lavanya Visvabharathy, Barbara Hanson, Zachary Orban, et al. Neuro-COVID long-haulers exhibit broad dysfunction in T cell memory generation and responses to vaccination. *medRxiv* (preprint) 2022. DOI:10.1101/2021.08.08.21261763.
- Matthew Walker. *Why We Sleep: The New Science of Sleep and Dreams.* London: Simon & Schuster, 2017.
- Gerd Wallukat, Bettina Hohberger, Katrin Wenzel, et al. Functional autoantibodies against G-protein coupled receptors in patients with persistent Long-COVID-19 symptoms. *Journal of Translational Autoimunity* 2021; 4: 100100.
- Xin Wang, Elena Gkrouzman, Danieli Andrade, et al. COVID-19 and antiphospholipid antibodies: a position statement and management guidance from Anti-Phospholipid Syndrome Alliance for Clinical Trials and InternatiOnal Networking (APS ACTION). *Lupus* 2021; 30: 2276–85.
- Stacey Weiner. 'Scary and confusing': When kids suffer from long COVID-19. *Association of American Medical Colleges News*, 9 December 2021. Available at https://www.aamc.org/news-insights/scary-and-confusing-when-kids-suffer-long-covid-19

- Leonard B Weinstock, Jill B Brook, Arthur S Walters, et al. Mast cell activation symptoms are prevalent in long-COVID. *International Journal of Infectious Diseases* 2021; 112: 217–26.
- Jan Wenzel, Josephine Lampe, Helge Müller-Fielitz, et al. The SARS-CoV-2 main protease Mpro causes microvascular brain pathology by cleaving NEMO in brain endothelial cells. *Nature Neuroscience* 2021; 24: 1522–33.
- Simon Wessely, Anthony David, Sue Butler, et al. Management of chronic (post-viral) fatigue syndrome. *Journal of the Royal College of GPs* 1989; 39: 26–29.
- P D White, K A Goldsmith, A L Johnson, et al. Comparison of adaptive pacing therapy, cognitive behaviour therapy, graded exercise therapy, and specialist medical care for chronic fatigue syndrome (PACE): a randomised trial. *The Lancet* 2011; 377: 823–36.
- Carolyn E Wilshire, Tom Kindlon, Robert Courtney, et al. Rethinking the treatment of chronic fatigue syndrome–a reanalysis and evaluation of findings from a recent major trial of graded exercise and CBT. *BMC Psychology* 2019; 6: 6.
- Lisa Winder. NIH grants $470 million for study of long COVID. *The Scientist*, 16 September 2021. Available at https://www.the-scientist.com/news-opinion/nih-grants-470-million-for-study-of-long-covid-69192
- Jamie Wood, Laura Tabacof, Jenna Tosto-Mancuso, et al. Levels of end-tidal carbon dioxide are low despite normal respiratory rate in individuals with long COVID. *Journal of Breath Research* 2021; 16: 017101.
- Yongjian Wu, Cheng Guo, Lantian Tang, et al. Prolonged presence of SARS-CoV-2 viral RNA in faecal samples. *The Lancet Gastroenterology & Hepatology* 2021; 5: 434–35.
- Yan Xie, Benjamin Bowe, Ziyad Al-Aly. Burdens of post-acute sequelae of COVID-19 by severity of acute infection,

demographics and health status. *Nature Communications* 2021; 12: 6571.

- Yan Xie, Evan Xu, Benjamin Bowe, et al. Long-term cardiovascular outcomes of COVID-19. *Nature Medicine* 2022; 28: 583–90.
- Masanori Yamato, Yosky Kataoka. Fatigue sensation following peripheral viral infection is triggered by neuroinflammation: who will answer these questions? *Neural Regeneration Research* 2015; 10: 203–04.
- Habib Yaribeygi, Yunes Panehi, Hedayay Sahraei, et al. The impact of stress on body function: a review. *EXCLI Journal* 2017; 16: 1057–72.
- John O Younge, Machteld F Wery, Rinske A Gotink, et al. Web-based mindfulness intervention in heart disease: a randomized controlled trial. *PLoS One* 2015; 10: e0143843.
- Jarred Younger, Luke Parkitny, David McLain. The use of low-dose naltrexone (LDN) as a novel anti-inflammatory treatment for chronic pain. *Clinical Rheumatology* 2014; 33: 451–59.
- Lanlan Zhang, Elizabeth A Reynolds Losin, Yoni K Ashar, et al. Gender biases in estimation of others' pain. *Journal of Pain* 2021; 22: 1048–59.
- Peixun Zhang, Jia Li, Huixin Liu, et al. Long-term bone and lung consequences associated with hospital-acquired severe acute respiratory syndrome: a 15-year follow-up from a prospective cohort study. *Bone Research* 2020; 8: 8.
- Andreas Zollner, Robert Koch, Almina Jukic, et al. Postacute COVID-19 is characterized by gut viral antigen persistence in inflammatory bowel diseases. *Gastroenterology* 2022. DOI:10.1053/j.gastro.2022.04.037.
- Yu Zuo, Shanea K Estes, Ramadan A Ali, et al. Prothrombotic autoantibodies in serum from patients hospitalized with COVID-19. *Science Translational Medicine* 2020; 12: eabd3876.

References

- Simeon J Zürcher, Céline Banzer, Christine Adamus, et al. Post-viral mental health sequelae in infected persons associated with COVID-19 and previous epidemics and pandemics: systematic review and meta-analysis of prevalence estimates. *Journal of Infection and Public Health* 2022; 15: 599–608.

Index

preprints, 199–202
see also medication
tremors, 52
triple therapy, 199–200
tryptophan, 96–7
Tuller, David, 125–6
tumours, 29, 69, 86, 186
Twitter, 30, 190, 219
type A personalities, 37

unconscious bias, 107
United Kingdom, 41, 43, 53, 62, 65,
    110–11, 184, 194
United States, 43, 47, 65, 111
United States Marine Corps, 234
University College London, 94, 189, 246
University of California, Berkeley, 126
University of Minnesota, 51
University of Oxford, 243–4
University of the Pacific, 166
urinary incontinence, 9
urinary symptoms, 52
uveitis, 217

vaccines, 11, 28, 41, 58, 63, 78, 137–8,
    180, 184
vagus nerve, 39, 40, 68, 82, 139, 173, 209–10
van der Kolk, Bessel, 231
vascular function impairment, 89–90
vasculitis, 99
ventilation, 28
vertigo, 52, 148
vicious cycles, 223
viral loads, 28
Virios Therapeutics, 248
viruses
    debris/persistence, 65, 75–84, 105,
        117, 194, 207, 223, 244, 245
    loads, 28
    reactivation, 25, 27, 65, 73–5, 174
    toxicity, 65

vision problems, 16
vitamins, 202, 208
vomiting, 52

Walker, Lucy, 153
Walker, Matthew, 135, 160
Ward, Lisa, 238
Watkins, Rhoda, 239
weight changes, 10, 52, 128
Weil, Andrew, 178
white blood cells, 27, 29, 51, 69, 98
    B cells, 27, 29, 69, 74, 95, 174, 186,
        216, 234, 242
    eosinophils, 201
    T cells, *see* T cells
Whittaker, Elizabeth, 57
Why We Sleep (Walker), 125, 160
WILCO project, 241
women, 23, 30–31, 45, 107–22
    autoimmunity and, 25–6, 99, 110
    chronic illnesses and, 109–11
    hormone replacement therapy, 108,
        206
    medically unexplained symptoms
        and, 111–15
    menstrual cycle, 9, 52, 108, 115–18,
        121
    pregnancy, 115
World Health Organization (WHO),
    11, 250

xenon gas, 103

Yale University, 245
yoga, 40, 140, 211, 226
YouTube, 2
Yu Zuo, 101

zinc, 209
ZOE app, 15, 31
Zofin, 247–8